The Hormone Code

Balancing Hormones for Weight Loss, Longevity, and Optimal Health

Alexandra Hart

Contents

Copyright	VI
About Alexandra Hart	1
About the Book	3
The Code Series	5
Introduction	11
Part I	18
1. Cortisol	19
2. Estrogen	37
3. Progesterone	57
4. Thyroid Hormones	69
Part II	82
5. Depression, Anxiety, and Hormonal Imbalance	83
6. The Gut-Hormone-Mind Connection	96
Part III	108
7. The Food We Eat and Its Impact on Hormonal Health	109
8. The Food Industry's Role in Hormonal Imbalance	119

9. The Sugar-Hormone Connection	130
Part IV	141
10. Exercise for Hormonal Health	142
11. Sleep and Hormones	152
12. Stress Reduction and Mindfulness for Hormone Balance	160
13. Toxins, Hormones, and Detoxification	169
Part V	181
14. Menstrual Cycle and Hormonal Fluctuations	182
15. Hormone Health and Skin, Hair, and Nails	191
16. Perimenopause and Menopause	201
17. Postpartum Hormonal Health	215
18. Hormonal Imbalances and Fertility	225
19. Addressing Common Myths About Hormonal Health	241
Conclusion	249
Glossary of Terms	259
Dear Reader,	262
Other Books by Alexandra Hart	263
About Alexandra Hart	265

Copyright © 2024 by Alexandra Hart

All rights reserved.

No portion of this book may be reproduced in any form without written permission from the publisher or author, except as permitted by U.S. copyright law.

About Alexandra Hart

Alexandra Hart is a dedicated psychiatrist with a passion for understanding the complexities of the human mind and fostering mental well-being. With years of experience in the field, Alexandra has worked extensively with individuals from diverse backgrounds, helping them navigate life's challenges and achieve emotional balance. Her approach to psychiatry is deeply rooted in empathy, evidence-based practices, and a commitment to holistic care.

Driven by a desire to make mental health resources accessible and relatable, Alexandra has contributed to various mental health initiatives and projects, sharing her insights on topics such as emotional resilience, personal growth, and the importance of self-care. Her work reflects a profound understanding of the interconnectedness of mental health, identity, and overall well-being.

In her free time, Alexandra enjoys exploring the arts, engaging in thoughtful discussions, and continuously learning about the ever-evolving field of psychiatry. She is passionate about helping others lead fulfilling lives and is dedicated to making a positive impact on the mental health landscape.

To read more books from the author and join her community, you can scan the code below, or go to the link – https://substack.com/@alexandrahart1

About the Book

ARE YOU STRUGGLING WITH stubborn weight gain, low energy, or hormonal imbalances? Unlock the secrets to lasting health and vitality with **"The Hormone Code: Balancing Hormones for Weight Loss, Longevity, and Optimal Health,"** the ultimate guide for women looking to regain control of their bodies and well-being through hormone balance.

Hormonal imbalances can wreak havoc on your metabolism, mood, and overall health—whether it's dealing with menopause, postpartum recovery, or navigating life after birth control. This comprehensive **hormone balance book** for women provides science-backed strategies to restore balance. Learn how your hormones—especially **progesterone, cortisol, and thyroid**—affect your body and how to reset them naturally. Through holistic solutions like a tailored **hormone-balanced diet** and lifestyle adjustments, you'll be empowered to take control of your health at any age.

Imagine feeling energetic, losing stubborn weight, and enjoying vibrant health for years to come. **"The Hormone Code"** gives you the tools to achieve this. Whether you're looking for answers to **hormone balance after menopause**, dealing with **hormone balance hair loss**, or seeking guidance for **hormone balance for women**

after birth control, this book will help you take actionable steps. It's the go-to **hormone balance bible** for those seeking solutions for weight loss, mental clarity, and longevity.

Don't wait to reclaim your health! Grab your copy of **"The Hormone Code: Balancing Hormones for Weight Loss, Longevity, and Optimal Health"** today. This **women's hormone balance book** will equip you with the knowledge and tools to feel your best, overcome hormonal imbalances, and live a life full of energy and confidence.

The Code Series

Dr. Alexandra Hart

Unlock the secrets to optimal health and well-being with *The Code Series*. This groundbreaking collection dives deep into the complex interplay between hormones, metabolism, and nutrition, offering readers practical strategies to transform their health through fasting, diet, and lifestyle changes. Each book in the series unpacks a vital aspect of health, providing easy-to-understand science-backed solutions for managing weight, boosting energy, and preventing disease. Whether you're struggling with insulin resistance, sugar addiction, or hormonal imbalances, *The Code Series* equips you with the tools to take control of your health and live a longer, more vibrant life.

The Insulin Code, the flagship book in the series, reveals how fasting can be the key to mastering insulin and metabolic health, while upcoming titles will continue to decode the critical factors that influence overall wellness.

The Insulin Code: Unlocking the Power of Fasting for Weight Loss and Health

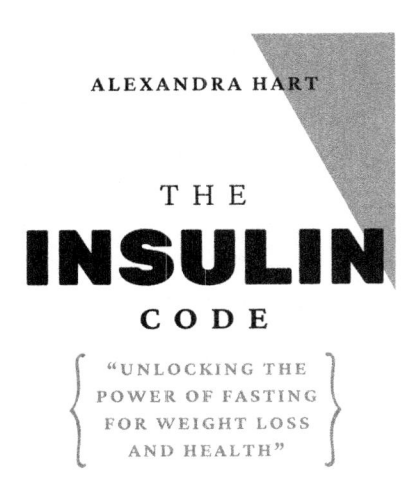

Are you struggling with weight gain, fatigue, or managing chronic conditions like type 2 diabetes? What if the key to reversing these issues isn't about restrictive diets, but lies in mastering your body's most important hormone—insulin?

The Insulin Code by Alexandra Hart reveals the science behind insulin and offers a powerful, natural solution: fasting.

In this insightful book, Alexandra Hart simplifies the complexities of insulin management, making it accessible for everyone. Learn how insulin plays a central role in fat storage, metabolism, and overall health, and how insulin resistance is the hidden cause of many chronic diseases. Discover how intermittent fasting can reset your insulin levels, promote fat-burning, and restore your metabolic health. Backed by science and personal stories, Hart provides practical fasting protocols, meal plans, and easy-to-follow strategies for lasting health transformation.

Picture a life where losing weight feels effortless, your energy levels soar, and chronic diseases like type 2 diabetes become manageable—or even reversible. Through practical advice and real-world success stories, **The Insulin Code** empowers you to take control of your health by using fasting to reset your metabolism, engage in autophagy (the body's natural detox and repair process), and regain the energy you've been missing.

Ready to break free from the cycle of insulin resistance and take back control of your health?

Start your journey with **The Insulin Code** today, and unlock the benefits of fasting and insulin management for sustainable, long-term well-being.

The Sugar Code: Breaking Free from Sugar Addiction for Better Health and Diabetes Control

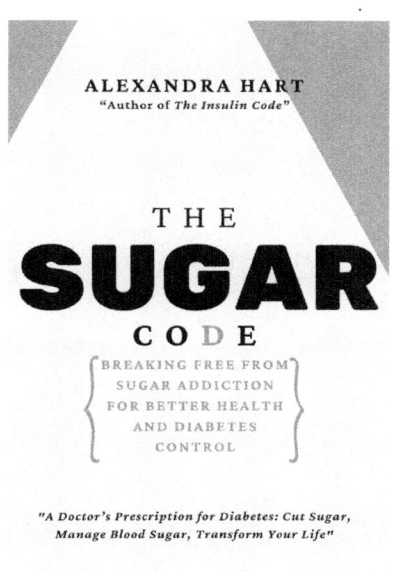

The Sugar Code

Are you caught in the cycle of sugar addiction and struggling to control your blood sugar? Does managing your diabetes feel like an uphill battle with no clear path to success?

Imagine living a life where your blood sugar is stable, your cravings are under control, and you have the tools to prevent or reverse diabetes. **The Sugar Code** is your guide to making that vision a reality. Whether you've been diagnosed with Type 2 diabetes or want to stop prediabetes in its tracks, this book will give you the actionable, science-based strategies you need.

The Sugar Code offers an evidence-based approach to managing insulin resistance and breaking free from the grip of sugar. The book covers the entire journey of diabetes control—from understanding how sugar impacts your body to practical steps you can take to reduce sugar, improve your insulin sensitivity, and regain control of your health. You'll find answers to the most pressing questions about diabetes and sugar, all explained in a clear, relatable way.

In this comprehensive guide, you'll discover:

- **The science behind sugar addiction**: Learn how sugar impacts brain chemistry and contributes to insulin resistance, and what you can do to manage cravings.

- **The critical role of insulin resistance** in diabetes and how reducing sugar can help reverse this condition.

- How **fructose** specifically worsens insulin resistance and liver health, contributing to the rise of diabetes.

- The **gut-brain-sugar connection**: Discover how sugar affects the gut microbiome and how restoring gut health can help control blood sugar.

- **Fasting protocols for diabetes management**: Learn about safe, effective fasting strategies that can help reset your metabolism and improve insulin function.

- **Meal plans and diabetes-friendly recipes**: Get sample meal plans and simple, delicious recipes that will help you reduce sugar while enjoying balanced nutrition.

- **Practical tools for tracking your progress**: A guide to using continuous glucose monitors (CGMs), blood glucose meters, and apps to track your blood sugar levels and optimize your insulin control.

Imagine a life where your diabetes is no longer in control. Visualize a future where your blood sugar is stable, your energy levels are consistent, and you're free from the highs and lows of sugar cravings. With **The Sugar Code**, you'll gain the knowledge and practical tools to reclaim your health. This book empowers you to make sustainable changes that improve insulin sensitivity, reduce sugar dependence, and prevent complications from diabetes.

- Feel confident with **science-backed strategies** that can help you reduce or even eliminate your need for medications.

- Learn how to break free from the **diet culture traps** and sugar myths that keep so many people stuck.

- Find practical, **step-by-step guidance** to take control of your blood sugar and live a healthier, more vibrant life.

Now is the time to take control of your diabetes and break the cycle of sugar addiction. **The Sugar Code** provides the tools, strategies, and scientific insights to transform your health and reverse the course of diabetes. Whether you're newly diagnosed or have been managing diabetes for years, this book will help you master your blood sugar and unlock a healthier future.

Start your journey to a diabetes-free life today by embracing the simple, powerful steps outlined in **The Sugar Code**.

Introduction

The Importance of Hormonal Balance for Women

Hormones are essential chemical messengers that play a crucial role in nearly every aspect of a woman's health. From regulating metabolism and energy levels to influencing mood and reproductive health, the balance of hormones like cortisol, estrogen, progesterone, and thyroid hormones is key to feeling your best. When these hormones are in harmony, the body functions optimally, and a woman can experience stable energy, a healthy weight, and mental clarity. However, when hormonal imbalances occur, the effects can be far-reaching, leading to weight gain, mood swings, fatigue, and long-term health issues.

In this chapter, we will explore the four key hormones that are central to a woman's health. We'll also highlight how hormonal imbalances can impact weight, metabolism, mental health, and longevity. Understanding these hormones and how they function is the first step toward reclaiming your health. Throughout the book, you will discover practical strategies and science-backed insights to help you balance your hormones and enhance your well-being.

The Key Hormones Affecting Women's Health

Hormones work together in complex systems to regulate essential functions in the body. For women, four hormones play especially important roles: **cortisol, estrogen, progesterone,** and **thyroid hormones**. Each of these hormones serves a unique function, but together they create a delicate balance that is critical to overall health. When any one of these hormones is out of balance, it can trigger a range of symptoms and health problems. Let's take a closer look at each of these hormones and how they influence a woman's body.

Cortisol: The Stress Hormone

Cortisol is produced by the adrenal glands and is commonly referred to as the "stress hormone" because it helps the body respond to stressful situations. It regulates the body's fight-or-flight response, which is critical for survival. Cortisol also plays a vital role in managing energy by breaking down fats and carbohydrates, controlling inflammation, and influencing blood pressure.

While cortisol is essential for short-term survival, chronic stress can cause cortisol levels to remain elevated for long periods. This constant state of high cortisol can have negative effects on the body, leading to weight gain, particularly around the abdomen, as well as fatigue, insomnia, and anxiety. Long-term elevation of cortisol levels can also lead to more serious health issues, such as insulin resistance, which increases the risk of weight gain and metabolic disorders.

The key to maintaining healthy cortisol levels lies in effective stress management. Relaxation techniques, adequate sleep, and balanced nutrition can help lower cortisol levels and promote overall hormonal health.

Estrogen: The Feminine Powerhouse

Estrogen is the primary female sex hormone and is responsible for the development and regulation of the female reproductive system. However, its role extends beyond reproduction. Estrogen influences a wide range of bodily functions, including bone density, cardiovascular health, skin health, and brain function. It also plays a significant role in metabolism and fat distribution.

When estrogen levels are balanced, the body can maintain healthy insulin sensitivity and regulate fat storage. However, imbalances in estrogen—whether too high or too low—can lead to various health issues. Estrogen dominance, or having too much estrogen relative to other hormones, is associated with weight gain, mood swings, and irregular menstrual cycles. On the other hand, low estrogen levels, which are common during perimenopause and menopause, can result in weight gain, hot flashes, and increased risk of osteoporosis.

Diet, exercise, and lifestyle choices all play a role in supporting healthy estrogen levels. In some cases, medical interventions such as hormone replacement therapy may be needed to restore balance.

Progesterone: The Calming Hormone

Progesterone is another key hormone in a woman's reproductive system. It works closely with estrogen to regulate the menstrual cycle and prepare the body for pregnancy. In addition to its role in reproduction, progesterone has a calming effect on the body. It promotes restful sleep, reduces anxiety, and helps balance the effects of estrogen.

Low progesterone levels can lead to a variety of symptoms, including anxiety, insomnia, and irregular menstrual cycles. Progesterone deficiency is also common during perimenopause, contributing to the hormonal imbalance that many women experience during this transition. Chronic stress can further suppress progesterone production, exacerbating these issues.

Balancing progesterone can often be achieved through natural means, such as reducing stress and adopting a nutrient-rich diet. Herbal supplements like Vitex (chasteberry) are also known to support healthy progesterone levels.

Thyroid Hormones: The Metabolic Regulators

The thyroid is a small gland located in the neck, and it produces hormones that regulate metabolism, energy levels, and body temperature. The thyroid produces two primary hormones, thyroxine (T4) and triiodothyronine (T3), both of which play a critical role in keeping the body's metabolism running efficiently.

When the thyroid is underactive, a condition known as hypothyroidism, metabolism slows down, leading to weight gain, fatigue, and depression. Conversely, an overactive thyroid, known as hyperthyroidism, speeds up metabolism, which can result in weight loss, anxiety, and heart palpitations.

Thyroid imbalances are particularly common in women, especially as they age or after pregnancy. Supporting thyroid function through a diet rich in iodine, selenium, and other key nutrients can help maintain balance. In cases of thyroid disorders, medical intervention such as hormone replacement therapy may be necessary.

The Widespread Impact of Hormonal Imbalance

The effects of hormonal imbalance can be far-reaching and profound. Hormones regulate many of the body's essential functions, so when they become imbalanced, the consequences are felt in various areas of health and well-being. The following sections provide a snapshot of how hormonal imbalances can affect women, particularly in the areas of weight, metabolism, mental health, and longevity.

1. Weight and Metabolism

Hormonal imbalances, particularly in cortisol, estrogen, and thyroid hormones, can significantly impact weight and metabolism. For instance, high levels of cortisol can lead to an increase in abdominal fat, while low levels of estrogen are associated with fat storage in the hips and thighs. Thyroid disorders can either slow or speed up metabolism, making it challenging to maintain a healthy weight.

Balancing these hormones is essential for restoring a healthy metabolism. Lifestyle changes such as a hormone-friendly diet, regular physical activity, and stress management can help regulate hormone levels and promote weight loss or weight maintenance.

2. Mental Health

Hormonal fluctuations have a direct impact on mental health. Elevated cortisol levels are associated with anxiety, irritability, and even depression. Similarly, low levels of estrogen, particularly during perimenopause and menopause, can lead to mood swings and cognitive decline. Thyroid imbalances are also a common cause of mood disorders, as low thyroid hormones affect the production of serotonin, a neurotransmitter that regulates mood.

Balancing hormones can significantly improve mental health, leading to more emotional stability and better cognitive function. Practices such as mindfulness, exercise, and ensuring adequate sleep are key to supporting both hormonal and mental well-being.

3. Longevity and Aging

Hormonal balance plays a pivotal role in how the body ages. Estrogen, for example, is protective against bone loss and supports cardiovascular health, while thyroid hormones keep metabolism functioning efficiently as the body ages. Cortisol, when kept in check, helps reduce chronic inflammation, which is a major contributor to aging and degenerative diseases.

By maintaining hormone balance, women can protect their long-term health, reduce the risk of age-related diseases, and enjoy a better quality of life as they age.

What to Expect from This Book

This book is designed to provide you with the knowledge and tools you need to understand your hormones and take control of your health. Each chapter will offer insights into how specific hormones function and how they affect your body, followed by practical strategies to help you restore balance. Throughout the book, you'll find evidence-based advice on nutrition, exercise, stress management, and natural remedies that support hormonal health.

Here's a preview of what you'll find in the coming chapters:

- **Comprehensive Understanding:** Each hormone will be explored in depth, helping you understand how it impacts your health and how you can achieve balance.

- **Actionable Strategies:** From dietary changes to lifestyle adjustments, each chapter will provide practical steps to support your hormone health.

- **Empowerment Through Knowledge:** You will be equipped with the information you need to make informed decisions about your health and take proactive steps toward better well-being.

By the end of this book, you will have a clear understanding of how to balance your hormones and take charge of your health. Whether you are dealing with weight issues, fatigue, or mood swings, you'll find the tools you need to restore harmony in your body and improve your overall well-being.

Part I

Understanding the Hormones

Chapter 1

Cortisol

The Stress Hormone

Cortisol is often described as the body's "primary stress hormone," yet its role extends far beyond mere stress response. Produced by the adrenal glands, cortisol is integral to numerous essential bodily functions. Its regulation is critical to maintaining homeostasis, and disturbances in cortisol levels—whether due to chronic stress, illness, or lifestyle factors—can lead to profound health issues. Understanding the normal, healthy functioning of cortisol in the body is key to recognizing when it becomes imbalanced.

In this chapter, we will delve into the physiological role of cortisol, how chronic stress disrupts its delicate balance, and the downstream effects of that imbalance, including weight gain and fatigue. Through this, you will gain an understanding of the body's complex relationship with cortisol and how to take proactive steps to maintain hormonal balance.

The Normal Function of Cortisol in the Body

While cortisol is best known for its involvement in the stress response, it is a vital hormone with a range of important functions in the body. Cortisol operates in a rhythmic pattern known as the circadian rhythm, peaking in the early morning to help the body wake up and gradually declining throughout the day to allow for rest and recovery. This daily cycle is crucial for maintaining energy levels, supporting metabolism, and regulating other key systems. Here's a closer look at the normal, healthy roles cortisol plays:

1. Energy Regulation and Glucose Metabolism

Cortisol is deeply involved in the regulation of glucose, the body's primary energy source. One of its primary roles is to ensure that the brain, muscles, and vital organs have enough glucose available, particularly during times of stress or fasting. Under normal conditions, cortisol stimulates the liver to convert stored glycogen into glucose, a process called **gluconeogenesis**. This ensures that blood sugar levels remain stable, preventing hypoglycemia (low blood sugar) between meals or during periods of intense activity.

By making glucose readily available, cortisol plays an essential role in preventing energy shortages that could impair critical functions such as cognition, muscle contraction, and organ function. In fact, without cortisol, the body would struggle to maintain adequate energy stores, particularly during fasting or strenuous physical exertion.

2. Fat and Protein Metabolism

In addition to its role in glucose regulation, cortisol facilitates the breakdown of fats and proteins. This is particularly important during periods of stress or fasting when the body needs to mobilize stored energy. Cortisol signals fat cells to release fatty acids into the bloodstream, which can then be used by muscles and other tissues as an alternative energy source to glucose. This process, called **lipolysis**, is a key component of maintaining energy balance during times of caloric restriction or increased demand.

Similarly, cortisol helps break down proteins into amino acids, which can be used to support tissue repair, immune function, and the production of enzymes and other molecules. In this way, cortisol ensures that the body has the building blocks it needs to function properly, even under challenging conditions.

3. Inflammatory Response and Immune Function

Cortisol also plays a critical role in regulating inflammation and immune function. In times of acute stress, cortisol acts as an anti-inflammatory agent, preventing the immune system from overreacting to injury or infection. This is an essential function, as unchecked inflammation can lead to tissue damage and contribute to a host of chronic diseases.

Under normal circumstances, cortisol helps modulate the immune response, keeping it in check and ensuring that inflammation is properly regulated. This is why cortisol is sometimes used medically in the form of corticosteroids to treat conditions characterized by excessive inflammation, such as autoimmune diseases or allergic reactions.

However, the anti-inflammatory effects of cortisol are a double-edged sword. While short-term cortisol release helps control inflammation, chronic overproduction of cortisol can suppress the immune system, making the body more susceptible to infections and impairing its ability to heal. Thus, while cortisol is essential for protecting the body from excessive inflammation, maintaining its balance is crucial for long-term immune health.

4. Blood Pressure and Cardiovascular Function

Cortisol also has a significant impact on cardiovascular health. It helps regulate blood pressure by influencing the body's retention of sodium and water. In stressful situations, cortisol helps maintain adequate blood pressure to ensure that vital organs receive sufficient blood flow and oxygen. This function is critical during the "fight-or-flight" response, when the body needs to ensure that muscles and the brain have the necessary resources to act quickly and efficiently.

In a healthy individual, cortisol levels return to normal once the stressor is removed, and blood pressure regulation resumes its normal state. However, prolonged elevation of cortisol, as seen in chronic stress, can contribute to sustained high blood pressure (hypertension), increasing the risk of cardiovascular diseases such as heart attacks and strokes.

5. Nervous System and Mood Regulation

Cortisol's influence extends to the nervous system, particularly in modulating mood, cognition, and emotional well-being. This hormone directly affects regions of the brain that regulate mood, such as the amygdala and hippocampus. When cortisol is released in response to acute stress, it enhances alertness, focus, and memory formation—functions that are critical when faced with a challenge or threat.

However, chronic stress and elevated cortisol levels can have the opposite effect. Long-term exposure to high cortisol can impair cognitive function, reduce memory retention, and contribute to mood disorders such as anxiety and depression. Research shows that elevated cortisol levels are often correlated with increased anxiety, irritability, and even long-term mental health issues like major depressive disorder.

How Chronic Stress Leads to Cortisol Imbalance and Weight Gain

The body's natural stress response is designed to be short-term. Once the stressful event has passed, cortisol levels should return to baseline, allowing the body to rest and recover. Unfortunately, in modern life, many of us face chronic stress—whether from work pressures, financial worries, or personal challenges—which leads to prolonged cortisol production. This persistent state of elevated cortisol disrupts the body's normal metabolic and hormonal processes, contributing to weight gain, especially in the abdominal area, as well as a host of other health issues.

1. Increased Abdominal Fat Storage

One of the most well-documented effects of chronic cortisol elevation is an increase in abdominal fat. Cortisol encourages the storage of visceral fat, the type of fat that surrounds internal organs in the abdominal cavity. This type of fat is particularly dangerous because it is metabolically active and releases pro-inflammatory substances, contributing to a higher risk of cardiovascular disease, diabetes, and metabolic syndrome.

The mechanism behind this fat storage is twofold:

- **Energy Conservation:** Cortisol promotes the storage of fat during stressful times to ensure that the body has a readily available energy reserve. While this may have been an adaptive response in our evolutionary past, when food scarcity was common, in the modern world—where stress is abundant, but food is readily available—it leads to excess fat accumulation.

- **Increased Appetite for High-Calorie Foods:** Cortisol increases cravings for high-calorie foods, particularly those rich in sugar and fat. This is because cortisol raises blood sugar levels, which subsequently triggers insulin release. Over time, this cycle can contribute to insulin resistance and make it harder for the body to metabolize glucose efficiently, leading to further fat accumulation.

2. Impact on Muscle Mass and Metabolism

Cortisol doesn't just promote fat storage; it can also break down muscle tissue. When cortisol is elevated for long periods, the body begins to catabolize muscle protein to provide glucose for energy through a process called **proteolysis**. The loss of muscle mass can slow down metabolism, as muscle is more metabolically active than fat. This can make weight gain more likely, even if calorie intake remains stable.

This muscle breakdown, combined with increased fat storage, leads to a decrease in the body's overall metabolic rate. A slower metabolism makes it increasingly difficult to lose weight and easier to gain it, creating a vicious cycle of weight gain and metabolic dysfunction.

3. Insulin Resistance and Metabolic Dysfunction

Chronic exposure to cortisol can interfere with the body's insulin sensitivity. Normally, insulin helps regulate blood sugar levels by facilitating the uptake of glucose into cells for energy production. However, elevated cortisol can cause cells to become less responsive to insulin, leading to **insulin resistance**. Over time, this condition can result in higher blood sugar levels, increased fat storage, and a greater risk of developing type 2 diabetes.

Cortisol-induced insulin resistance also makes it more challenging to lose weight, as the body becomes more efficient at storing, rather than burning, calories. This metabolic dysfunction is a key factor in the development of obesity and other related conditions.

Symptoms of Cortisol Imbalance

Recognizing the signs of cortisol imbalance is critical for identifying when chronic stress is taking a toll on your health. The most common symptoms of cortisol dysregulation include:

1. Fatigue

Despite cortisol's role in boosting energy during times of stress, prolonged elevation often leads to the opposite effect—chronic fatigue. This happens because the body's energy reserves become depleted over time, leading to persistent feelings of tiredness even after adequate sleep.

2. Sleep Disturbances

Cortisol follows a diurnal rhythm, peaking in the morning and gradually declining throughout the day. Chronic stress can disrupt this rhythm, leading to elevated cortisol levels at night, making it difficult to fall asleep or stay asleep.

3. Weight Gain, Especially Around the Abdomen

As noted, one of the most visible signs of cortisol imbalance is the accumulation of fat around the abdomen. This type of fat is particularly resistant to diet and exercise and poses serious health risks.

4. Frequent Illness and Poor Immune Function

Prolonged cortisol elevation suppresses the immune system, increasing susceptibility to infections and slowing recovery from illness.

Chronic stress weakens the body's ability to fend off viruses and bacteria, leaving individuals vulnerable to frequent colds, infections, and other illnesses.

5. Anxiety, Irritability, and Mood Swings

Cortisol's impact on brain function is profound. High levels of cortisol are associated with increased anxiety, irritability, and emotional instability. In the long term, chronic cortisol elevation can contribute to serious mental health conditions such as depression.

6. Cognitive Impairment

Cortisol can affect memory and concentration by damaging the hippocampus, the part of the brain responsible for forming new memories. Over time, this can lead to difficulty focusing, forgetfulness, and cognitive decline.

The Link Between Cortisol and Insulin Resistance

Cortisol and insulin are two of the most critical hormones for regulating metabolism, and their relationship plays a significant role in your overall health. While both hormones are essential for normal bodily functions, chronic stress and the resulting sustained elevation of cortisol levels can lead to insulin resistance, which increases the risk of weight gain, metabolic syndrome, and type 2 diabetes.

Understanding the Connection Between Cortisol and Insulin

Cortisol, often referred to as the "stress hormone," is released by the adrenal glands in response to stress. One of its primary functions is to increase blood glucose levels by stimulating gluconeogenesis— the process where the liver produces glucose from non-carbohydrate sources like amino acids and fats. This increase in glucose provides immediate energy to help you cope with stress. Normally, once the stressful situation passes, cortisol levels decrease, and the body returns to its normal metabolic state.

Insulin, on the other hand, is produced by the pancreas and is responsible for regulating blood sugar levels by facilitating the uptake of glucose into cells, where it can be used for energy. When functioning properly, insulin ensures that glucose is effectively utilized by cells and helps maintain stable blood sugar levels.

However, when cortisol levels remain elevated over long periods due to chronic stress, this delicate balance between cortisol and insulin is disrupted. Persistent high levels of cortisol signal the body to continually produce glucose, leading to higher blood sugar levels. This constant demand for insulin to manage elevated blood glucose can cause the body's cells to become less sensitive to insulin—a condition known as **insulin resistance**.

How Chronic Cortisol Elevation Leads to Insulin Resistance

When cortisol remains elevated over time, several mechanisms come into play that increase the risk of insulin resistance:

1. **Continuous Glucose Production:** Under chronic stress, the liver is constantly stimulated to release glucose, even in the absence of immediate energy demands. This ongoing process leads to persistently elevated blood sugar levels, which forces the pancreas to produce more insulin to move glucose into cells. Over time, the cells of the body, particularly those in muscle and fat tissue, begin to resist insulin's signals, resulting in insulin resistance.

2. **Increased Visceral Fat Accumulation:** Cortisol promotes the storage of fat, particularly around the abdomen, which is known as visceral fat. This type of fat is metabolically active and releases inflammatory molecules that further impair insulin sensitivity. Visceral fat is closely linked with insulin resistance, and the more cortisol you produce, the more likely you are to accumulate this harmful fat, exacerbating insulin resistance.

3. **Impairment of Insulin Signaling Pathways:** Cortisol directly interferes with insulin signaling pathways at the cellular level. This impairs insulin's ability to effectively promote glucose uptake into cells, forcing the pancreas to produce even more insulin to overcome this resistance. Over time, the pancreas may struggle to keep up with the demand, leading to persistently high blood sugar levels and, eventually, the development of type 2 diabetes.

4. **Reduced Muscle Mass:** Chronic cortisol elevation can also contribute to the breakdown of muscle tissue to supply glucose through a process called proteolysis. Muscle tissue is an essential site for glucose uptake, and a reduction in muscle mass diminishes the body's ability to regulate blood sugar efficiently. As muscle mass declines, the risk of insulin resistance increases.

The Vicious Cycle of Cortisol and Insulin Resistance

Once insulin resistance sets in, a vicious cycle can develop. As the body becomes less responsive to insulin, the pancreas produces more of it to compensate. High insulin levels, in turn, promote fat storage, especially in the abdominal area, which exacerbates cortisol production and further fuels insulin resistance. This cycle can lead to metabolic syndrome, a cluster of conditions that includes high blood pressure, elevated blood sugar, excess body fat around the waist, and abnormal cholesterol levels.

The good news is that breaking this cycle is possible. By managing cortisol levels and improving insulin sensitivity, you can significantly reduce the risk of developing insulin resistance and related metabolic disorders.

Research Highlight: The Long-Term Effects of Chronic Cortisol Elevation on Brain Function, Mental Health, and Energy Levels

Chronic stress and the subsequent elevation of cortisol not only affect your metabolism but also have profound effects on your brain, mental health, and energy levels. While acute cortisol spikes during stress can enhance focus and energy in the short term, prolonged exposure to elevated cortisol can have detrimental effects on brain function, cognitive health, and emotional well-being.

1. Effects on Brain Function and Memory

Research has shown that long-term exposure to elevated cortisol levels can cause structural changes in the brain, particularly in the **hippocampus**, the region responsible for learning and memory. Cortisol disrupts the communication between neurons in the hippocampus, impairing memory formation and retrieval. Studies have demonstrated that individuals with chronically high cortisol levels often experience difficulties with memory, concentration, and decision-making.

In severe cases, chronic cortisol elevation can lead to shrinkage of the hippocampus, which is also associated with cognitive decline and an increased risk of developing neurodegenerative diseases such as Alzheimer's. These findings underscore the importance of maintaining healthy cortisol levels to protect cognitive function as we age.

2. Impact on Mental Health: Anxiety and Depression

Cortisol's influence on the **amygdala**, the brain's emotional center, also plays a significant role in mental health. Prolonged exposure to elevated cortisol levels has been linked to heightened anxiety, irritability, and mood swings. Cortisol affects the balance of neurotransmitters, including serotonin and dopamine, which are critical for regulating mood. When cortisol levels remain elevated for long periods, it can lead to an imbalance in these neurotransmitters, contributing to symptoms of anxiety and depression.

Studies have consistently shown that individuals with chronic stress and elevated cortisol are at a higher risk of developing mood disorders. For example, research published in the journal *Psychoneuroendocrinology* found that people with chronic stress exhibited both higher cortisol levels and a greater prevalence of depression and anxiety symptoms.

3. Effects on Energy Levels and Chronic Fatigue

Cortisol plays a key role in regulating energy levels throughout the day. Under normal conditions, cortisol follows a diurnal rhythm, peaking in the morning to provide a burst of energy and gradually declining by evening to support restful sleep. However, chronic stress can disrupt this rhythm, leading to consistently elevated cortisol levels, particularly in the evening when they should be low.

This disruption often leads to feelings of **chronic fatigue**, even after a full night's rest. Elevated evening cortisol can interfere with sleep quality, making it difficult to fall asleep or stay asleep. Over time, poor sleep contributes to further cortisol dysregulation, creating a cycle of exhaustion, stress, and elevated cortisol. Chronic fatigue syndrome and burnout are common consequences of long-term cortisol imbalance, as the body struggles to maintain energy levels in the face of persistent stress.

4. Neuroplasticity and Brain Resilience

One of the most concerning findings from research on cortisol and brain health is its negative impact on **neuroplasticity**, the brain's ability to adapt, grow, and recover from damage. Neuroplasticity is essential for learning, memory, and emotional resilience. Studies have shown that chronic cortisol elevation reduces the brain's capacity for neuroplasticity, making it more difficult to recover from stress, trauma, or injury.

However, it's important to note that the brain has remarkable regenerative abilities, and with proper stress management techniques, neuroplasticity can be preserved and even restored. This makes managing cortisol not only a priority for mental health but also for maintaining long-term cognitive resilience.

Practical Tips for Managing Stress and Lowering Cortisol

Given the wide-reaching effects of cortisol on metabolism, brain function, and overall health, managing cortisol levels is essential for maintaining both physical and mental well-being. Fortunately, there are many effective strategies for reducing cortisol and mitigating the impact of chronic stress. These approaches are simple yet powerful tools that can help you regain control over your body's stress response and promote hormonal balance.

1. Meditation and Mindfulness

Meditation has been extensively studied for its ability to reduce cortisol and promote relaxation. Research shows that practicing meditation regularly, even for as little as 10-15 minutes a day, can significantly lower cortisol levels. Meditation works by activating the parasympathetic nervous system, which counteracts the body's stress response, promoting relaxation and restoring balance.

Mindfulness, a type of meditation that focuses on staying present in the moment, is particularly effective for managing stress. Studies have shown that mindfulness-based stress reduction (MBSR) programs can lead to significant reductions in cortisol levels and improve overall well-being. By incorporating mindfulness into your daily routine, you can effectively reduce stress, improve focus, and enhance emotional regulation.

2. Deep Breathing Techniques

Deep breathing exercises are another simple yet highly effective way to lower cortisol levels. When you engage in deep, diaphragmatic breathing, you stimulate the body's relaxation response, which helps lower cortisol and reduce stress. The act of slowing down your breath sends signals to the brain to activate the parasympathetic nervous system, promoting a sense of calm and well-being.

A common technique is **4-7-8 breathing**, where you inhale deeply for four seconds, hold the breath for seven seconds, and exhale slowly for eight seconds. Practicing this technique for just a few minutes each day can have profound effects on cortisol levels, reducing stress and promoting relaxation.

3. Adaptogenic Herbs

Adaptogens are a class of herbs that help the body adapt to stress and normalize physiological processes. Several adaptogens have been shown to specifically target cortisol levels and help restore balance. Some of the most well-researched adaptogens for managing cortisol include:

- **Ashwagandha:** This adaptogen has been shown to reduce cortisol levels significantly in people experiencing chronic stress. A study published in the *Indian Journal of Psychological Medicine* found that ashwagandha supplementation reduced cortisol levels by up to 30%, while also improving stress resilience and overall well-being.

- **Rhodiola Rosea:** Known for its ability to enhance mental clarity and reduce fatigue, rhodiola has also been shown to lower cortisol and promote a more balanced stress response.

- **Holy Basil (Tulsi):** Traditionally used in Ayurvedic medicine, holy basil has been found to reduce anxiety, lower cortisol levels, and improve overall stress management.

Incorporating these herbs into your daily routine can support your body's natural stress response and help lower cortisol levels over time.

4. Prioritize Sleep

Sleep is one of the most powerful regulators of cortisol. A consistent sleep schedule, where you aim for 7-9 hours of sleep per night, is crucial for maintaining healthy cortisol rhythms. Avoiding stimulants like caffeine and reducing screen time before bed can also improve sleep quality and help lower nighttime cortisol levels.

5. Physical Activity

Regular physical activity is an effective way to manage stress and reduce cortisol levels. However, it's important to strike a balance—while moderate exercise like walking, yoga, or swimming can lower cortisol, overly intense workouts can raise cortisol levels in the short term. Engaging in activities that you enjoy and that promote relaxation, rather than pushing your body to its limits, will yield the best results for managing stress and cortisol.

By understanding the intricate relationship between cortisol and insulin resistance, as well as the long-term effects of elevated cortisol on brain function, mental health, and energy levels, you can take proactive steps to lower stress and regain control of your hormonal health. Implementing these practical tips—such as meditation, deep breathing, and incorporating adaptogens—will empower you to manage cortisol levels effectively and improve your overall well-being.

Chapter 2

Estrogen

The Feminine Powerhouse

Estrogen is often referred to as the "feminine hormone," but its influence goes well beyond regulating reproductive functions. This vital hormone impacts a range of bodily processes that are critical to a woman's health, including maintaining a healthy weight, ensuring mental clarity, and supporting emotional stability. From the onset of puberty through to menopause, estrogen is central to many aspects of physical and mental well-being.

In this chapter, we will explore the crucial role estrogen plays in reproductive health, weight management, and mental well-being. We will also examine how imbalances in estrogen—whether it is too high or too low—can disrupt a woman's health, leading to conditions like premenstrual syndrome (PMS), polycystic ovary syndrome (PCOS), and menopause-related symptoms. Understanding how estrogen affects various aspects of health is the first step in taking control of hormonal balance.

The Role of Estrogen in Reproductive Health

Estrogen is the principal hormone responsible for developing and regulating the female reproductive system. Produced primarily in the ovaries, estrogen is also synthesized in smaller amounts by the adrenal glands and fat tissue. Its levels naturally fluctuate throughout a woman's life, rising and falling during key reproductive phases like puberty, the menstrual cycle, pregnancy, and menopause.

1. Puberty and Sexual Maturation

During puberty, estrogen is responsible for the development of secondary sexual characteristics, such as breast growth, the widening of the hips, and the appearance of body hair. It also plays a key role in the maturation of the reproductive organs, including the uterus and ovaries, and in regulating the menstrual cycle.

Estrogen's role in the menstrual cycle is critical. In the first half of the cycle, during the **follicular phase**, estrogen levels increase, stimulating the thickening of the uterine lining (endometrium) in preparation for a possible pregnancy. Estrogen also promotes the growth and maturation of ovarian follicles, one of which will release an egg during ovulation. After ovulation, estrogen works alongside progesterone to maintain the uterine lining, ensuring that the body is ready for either pregnancy or menstruation.

2. Pregnancy and Childbearing

Estrogen continues to play an essential role during pregnancy. It regulates the development of the placenta and fetus, stimulates the growth of milk ducts in preparation for breastfeeding, and supports the expansion of the uterus as the baby grows. Moreover, estrogen helps maintain pregnancy by ensuring proper blood flow to the uterus and supporting the growth of the uterine lining, providing a stable environment for the fetus.

3. Menopause

As women approach menopause, estrogen levels begin to decline, leading to significant hormonal shifts. This transition often results in a range of symptoms, including hot flashes, night sweats, and mood changes, as the body adjusts to lower estrogen levels. Estrogen is also crucial for maintaining bone density, and its decline during menopause increases the risk of **osteoporosis**—a condition characterized by weakened bones and a higher likelihood of fractures.

Estrogen's Connection to Insulin Sensitivity and Fat Distribution

Estrogen's impact on health extends far beyond reproduction. One of its key roles is in regulating **insulin sensitivity** and **fat distribution**, both of which are crucial for metabolic health.

Insulin is the hormone responsible for controlling blood sugar levels by facilitating the uptake of glucose into cells, where it is used for energy. When cells become less sensitive to insulin—a condition known as **insulin resistance**—glucose remains in the bloodstream, which can elevate blood sugar levels and lead to weight gain, particularly in the abdominal area. Insulin resistance is a significant risk factor for type 2 diabetes and cardiovascular disease.

Estrogen's Role in Insulin Sensitivity

Estrogen plays a protective role in insulin sensitivity, especially during a woman's reproductive years. It enhances the body's ability to use insulin effectively by influencing metabolic pathways in the following ways:

- **Glucose Metabolism**: Estrogen improves how cells take up glucose and use it for energy. It increases the responsiveness of **insulin receptors** on cells, ensuring that glucose is absorbed efficiently. This prevents excessive sugar from circulating in the blood, which could otherwise contribute to weight gain and insulin resistance.

- **Fat Storage and Use**: Estrogen regulates how the body stores and uses fat. It encourages the accumulation of **subcutaneous fat**—fat stored just beneath the skin, particularly in the hips, thighs, and buttocks—which is considered metabolically healthier than **visceral fat** (fat stored around internal organs). Visceral fat is strongly linked to insulin resistance, heart disease, and metabolic syndrome.

During the reproductive years, estrogen promotes fat storage patterns that are beneficial for fertility and overall health. However, fluctuations in estrogen levels—whether during the menstrual cycle or in later stages of life—can significantly alter insulin sensitivity and fat distribution.

The Impact of Estrogen Deficiency on Insulin Sensitivity

As women age, particularly during **perimenopause** and **menopause**, estrogen levels naturally decline. The reduction of estrogen diminishes its protective effects on insulin sensitivity, leading to several metabolic changes:

- **Decreased Insulin Sensitivity**: Without estrogen's protective influence, the body becomes less efficient at utilizing insulin, which can lead to insulin resistance. As a result, higher levels of insulin are required to maintain normal blood sugar levels, increasing the risk of developing type 2 diabetes.

- **Shift in Fat Distribution**: Lower estrogen levels cause a shift in fat storage from the hips and thighs to the **abdominal area**, where fat tends to accumulate as **visceral fat**. This type of fat is more difficult to lose and is associated with a higher risk of metabolic diseases, including heart disease and insulin resistance.

- **Weight Gain**: Many women experience weight gain during menopause, despite no significant changes in diet or physical activity. This is largely due to the decline in estrogen's effects on metabolism, fat distribution, and insulin sensitivity.

Estrogen's Influence on Mental Well-Being

Estrogen plays a profound role in **mental health** and **cognitive function**, primarily through its connection to neurotransmitters such as **serotonin** and **dopamine**. These chemicals are essential for regulating mood, emotions, and cognitive processes. During a woman's reproductive years, estrogen helps stabilize neurotransmitter levels, promoting emotional balance and mental clarity.

How Estrogen Affects Serotonin Levels

Serotonin is often called the "feel-good" neurotransmitter because it helps regulate mood, contributes to a sense of well-being, and supports emotional stability. Estrogen affects serotonin production and function in several important ways:

- **Increased Serotonin Production**: Estrogen stimulates the production of serotonin by enhancing the activity of **tryptophan hydroxylase**, the enzyme responsible for converting the amino acid tryptophan into serotonin. When estrogen levels are optimal, serotonin production increases, leading to improved mood and emotional regulation.

- **Improved Serotonin Receptor Sensitivity**: Estrogen also boosts the sensitivity of **serotonin receptors**, enabling serotonin to bind more effectively and enhance its mood-stabilizing effects.

- **Reduced Breakdown of Serotonin**: Estrogen inhibits **monoamine oxidase (MAO)**, the enzyme that breaks down serotonin. This results in higher levels of serotonin in the brain, contributing to a calming, mood-stabilizing effect.

The Decline of Estrogen and Its Impact on Mood

Fluctuations in estrogen levels—such as during the menstrual cycle, pregnancy, or menopause—can cause significant shifts in mood, as serotonin levels also rise and fall.

- **Premenstrual Syndrome (PMS)**: In the days leading up to menstruation, estrogen levels drop, leading to a corresponding decline in serotonin levels. This often results in mood swings, irritability, and feelings of anxiety or sadness.

- **Perimenopause and Menopause**: As women approach menopause, estrogen levels fluctuate and eventually decline. This drop in estrogen can reduce serotonin production and receptor sensitivity, contributing to symptoms such as depression, anxiety, irritability, and mood swings.

- **Postpartum Depression**: After childbirth, estrogen levels drop rapidly, which can contribute to postpartum depression. This dramatic decline, combined with the physical and emotional demands of caring for a newborn, can significantly impact a woman's mood and mental health.

Cognitive Function and Brain Health

Beyond mood regulation, estrogen has a protective effect on **cognitive function**. Estrogen promotes **neuroplasticity**—the brain's ability to adapt, learn, and form new neural connections. Studies show that estrogen supports neuron health, reduces brain inflammation, and may even lower the risk of developing neurodegenerative diseases such as Alzheimer's.

Estrogen is particularly beneficial for the **hippocampus**, the brain region responsible for memory and learning. As estrogen levels decline during menopause, many women report experiencing **brain fog** or difficulty concentrating. These cognitive changes may be linked to the loss of estrogen's neuroprotective effects.

How Estrogen Imbalance Affects Women's Health

Estrogen imbalance—whether from estrogen dominance or deficiency—can have a range of effects on a woman's health. Let's examine how these conditions manifest and what symptoms women may experience.

1. Estrogen Dominance

Estrogen dominance occurs when estrogen levels are high relative to other hormones, particularly **progesterone**. This condition can be caused by factors such as exposure to estrogen-mimicking chemicals, obesity (as fat tissue produces estrogen), or a deficiency in progesterone.

Symptoms of estrogen dominance include:
- **Severe PMS**: High estrogen levels can worsen PMS symp-

toms like mood swings, bloating, and breast tenderness.

- **Polycystic Ovary Syndrome (PCOS)**: Women with PCOS may have elevated estrogen and androgen levels, which can lead to irregular periods, acne, and weight gain.

- **Weight Gain**: Estrogen dominance encourages fat storage in the hips and thighs, making weight loss more challenging.

- **Increased Cancer Risk**: Prolonged exposure to high estrogen levels increases the risk of estrogen-dependent cancers, such as breast and endometrial cancer.

2. Estrogen Deficiency

Estrogen deficiency is most common during perimenopause and menopause but can also occur in younger women due to excessive exercise, eating disorders, or certain medical conditions.

Symptoms of estrogen deficiency include:

- **Hot Flashes and Night Sweats**: One of the hallmark symptoms of low estrogen during menopause is sudden heat flashes that can disrupt sleep.

- **Mood Swings and Depression**: Low estrogen can cause a decline in serotonin, leading to mood swings, irritability, and depression.

- **Weight Gain**: Lower estrogen levels often lead to increased abdominal fat and a higher risk of metabolic syndrome.

- **Bone Loss (Osteoporosis)**: Estrogen is crucial for maintaining bone density, and its decline during menopause increases the risk of osteoporosis and fractures.

Estrogen's Connection to Insulin Sensitivity and Fat Distribution

Estrogen is a critical hormone that plays a central role in regulating not only reproductive health but also metabolic processes like insulin sensitivity and fat distribution. When we talk about insulin sensitivity, we're referring to how effectively the cells in your body respond to insulin, the hormone responsible for allowing glucose (sugar) to enter your cells to be used as energy. Estrogen has a protective effect on insulin sensitivity, which helps regulate blood sugar levels and prevent insulin resistance. Insulin resistance is a condition where the body's cells stop responding properly to insulin, leading to elevated blood sugar levels, weight gain, and an increased risk of type 2 diabetes and cardiovascular disease.

How Estrogen Influences Insulin Sensitivity

During a woman's reproductive years, estrogen helps maintain a healthy metabolism by improving insulin sensitivity. Estrogen acts on the insulin receptors in muscle and fat cells, making them more responsive to insulin's signals. This ensures that glucose is efficiently absorbed from the bloodstream into cells where it can be used for energy. This action helps keep blood sugar levels stable and prevents excess glucose from being stored as fat.

1. **Glucose Metabolism**: Estrogen enhances how cells metabolize glucose. It encourages muscle and fat cells to efficiently take up glucose from the bloodstream, thus preventing a buildup of blood sugar and reducing the risk of developing insulin resistance. Women with optimal estrogen levels often have an easier time maintaining a stable weight, as their bodies are better equipped to handle glucose.

2. **Fat Storage and Distribution**: Estrogen also plays a significant role in how and where the body stores fat. During the reproductive years, estrogen encourages the storage of **subcutaneous fat**—the fat located just beneath the skin—in areas such as the hips, thighs, and buttocks. This type of fat distribution is not only considered healthier but also serves an evolutionary purpose, as it supports fertility. Subcutaneous fat is less metabolically active than **visceral fat**, which accumulates around the organs in the abdominal region and is strongly linked to insulin resistance, heart disease, and inflammation.

When estrogen levels decline—such as during menopause—the body undergoes a metabolic shift. Fat storage patterns change, and women tend to store more fat in the abdominal region. This shift towards visceral fat not only contributes to changes in body shape but also carries significant health risks, as visceral fat is more likely to cause metabolic disturbances and increase the risk of chronic diseases.

Estrogen Deficiency and Insulin Resistance

As women age and enter perimenopause and menopause, their estrogen levels begin to drop. This decline in estrogen has a direct impact on insulin sensitivity:

1. **Decreased Insulin Sensitivity**: Without estrogen's protective effect, the body becomes less efficient at using insulin. As a result, more insulin is required to move glucose from the blood into cells, leading to **insulin resistance**. This means that despite normal or elevated insulin levels, cells are less responsive, causing blood sugar to remain elevated. Over time, this condition can progress to type 2 diabetes.

2. **Shift in Fat Distribution**: With lower estrogen levels, fat distribution shifts from the hips and thighs to the abdominal area, increasing the accumulation of visceral fat. This type of fat is more metabolically active and associated with insulin resistance, which makes weight gain more likely during menopause, even when diet and exercise remain consistent.

3. **Weight Gain**: Many women experience weight gain during menopause despite no significant changes in lifestyle. This is primarily due to the loss of estrogen's influence on metabolism, fat distribution, and insulin sensitivity. The decline in

estrogen levels can slow down metabolism, making it harder to lose weight and easier to store fat, particularly around the midsection.

The changes in body composition and metabolism during menopause can feel frustrating, but understanding how estrogen interacts with insulin and fat storage provides insight into how to manage these changes through diet, lifestyle adjustments, and hormonal support.

Research Highlight: The Relationship Between Estrogen and Serotonin (How It Impacts Mood and Brain Health)

Estrogen is often thought of as a hormone that primarily affects reproductive health, but its role in brain function and mood regulation is just as crucial. One of the most significant ways estrogen impacts the brain is through its interaction with **serotonin**, a neurotransmitter that plays a key role in regulating mood, emotions, and overall brain health. Serotonin is commonly known as the "feel-good" neurotransmitter because it promotes a sense of well-being and emotional balance.

How Estrogen Influences Serotonin

Estrogen's influence on serotonin is multifaceted. It impacts serotonin production, receptor sensitivity, and breakdown, which collectively contribute to mood stability and cognitive function.

1. **Increased Serotonin Production**: Estrogen stimulates the production of serotonin by increasing the activity of the enzyme tryptophan hydroxylase, which converts the amino acid tryptophan into serotonin in the brain. When estrogen levels are high—such as during the follicular phase of the menstrual cycle or during pregnancy—serotonin production increases, promoting a stable, positive mood.

2. **Improved Serotonin Receptor Sensitivity**: Estrogen enhances the sensitivity of **serotonin receptors**, making the brain more responsive to serotonin. This means that serotonin can more easily bind to its receptors, amplifying its mood-enhancing effects. Women with optimal estrogen levels often experience more emotional stability and resilience to stress.

3. **Reduced Breakdown of Serotonin**: Estrogen also reduces the breakdown of serotonin by inhibiting the enzyme **monoamine oxidase (MAO)**, which is responsible for degrading serotonin. By slowing down the breakdown process, estrogen ensures that serotonin remains active in the brain for longer, contributing to a sustained positive mood.

The Decline of Estrogen and Its Impact on Mood

When estrogen levels fluctuate or decline, as they do during the menstrual cycle, pregnancy, postpartum, and menopause, serotonin levels can also be affected. This connection between estrogen and serotonin is why many women experience mood changes during times of hormonal transition.

1. **Premenstrual Syndrome (PMS)**: In the days leading up to menstruation, estrogen levels drop, leading to a corresponding decline in serotonin levels. This reduction in serotonin is one of the primary reasons women experience mood swings, irritability, and feelings of anxiety or sadness before their period. This fluctuation in serotonin, combined with other hormonal changes, contributes to the emotional and psychological symptoms of PMS.

2. **Menopause**: During perimenopause and menopause, as estrogen levels decline significantly, serotonin production and receptor sensitivity are reduced. Many women in this phase of life report experiencing **depression, anxiety, irritability**, and **mood swings**—symptoms closely linked to changes in serotonin levels. The decline in serotonin may also contribute to the cognitive symptoms often reported during menopause, such as difficulty concentrating and memory issues.

3. **Postpartum Depression**: After childbirth, estrogen levels drop dramatically, which can have a significant impact on serotonin production and mood regulation. This sudden hormonal shift is one of the factors contributing to

postpartum depression, a condition that affects many new mothers. The combination of a steep drop in estrogen and the demands of caring for a newborn can lead to mood disturbances, anxiety, and depression.

Estrogen's Role in Cognitive Function and Brain Health

In addition to mood regulation, estrogen plays a critical role in maintaining **cognitive function** and **brain health**. Estrogen promotes **neuroplasticity**, the brain's ability to form new connections and adapt to new information. This is essential for learning, memory, and overall cognitive resilience.

1. **Memory and Learning**: Estrogen supports the health of neurons, particularly in the **hippocampus**, a region of the brain that is crucial for memory formation and spatial navigation. Research shows that women tend to perform better on memory and cognitive tasks during the high-estrogen phase of their menstrual cycle.

2. **Neuroprotection**: Estrogen also has **anti-inflammatory** effects in the brain, helping to reduce the risk of neurodegenerative diseases such as Alzheimer's disease. It promotes the growth and survival of neurons and may protect against age-related cognitive decline. This is why many women report experiencing **"brain fog"** or difficulty concentrating as their estrogen levels decline during menopause, as the loss of estrogen's neuroprotective effects becomes more evident.

Dietary and Lifestyle Strategies to Regulate Estrogen Levels

Maintaining balanced estrogen levels is crucial for both metabolic health and mental well-being. While hormone replacement therapy (HRT) can be an option for some women, there are also natural, non-pharmaceutical strategies that can help regulate estrogen levels through diet, exercise, and detoxification.

1. Phytoestrogens

Phytoestrogens are plant compounds that mimic the effects of estrogen in the body. These naturally occurring substances can bind to estrogen receptors and exert a mild estrogenic effect, which can help support hormone balance, especially during menopause when estrogen levels are low.

- **Flaxseeds**: Flaxseeds are rich in **lignans**, a type of phytoestrogen that can help balance estrogen levels by either enhancing or moderating the hormone's effects. Ground flaxseeds can be easily added to smoothies, oatmeal, or salads for an estrogen boost.

- **Soy**: Soy products, such as tofu, tempeh, and edamame, contain **isoflavones**, another potent type of phytoestrogen. Studies have shown that soy consumption may help alleviate some symptoms of low estrogen, such as hot flashes and night sweats, and may support heart and bone health.

- **Legumes**: Lentils, chickpeas, and beans also contain phytoestrogens and can be incorporated into the diet to help regulate estrogen levels.

For women with estrogen dominance, phytoestrogens can help by competing with the body's own estrogen for receptor sites, thereby reducing the overall estrogenic effect. Conversely, for women with low estrogen, phytoestrogens can provide a gentle, estrogen-like effect, alleviating symptoms of estrogen deficiency.

2. Exercise

Regular physical activity is one of the most effective ways to support estrogen balance. Exercise helps regulate estrogen production, reduce body fat (which is a source of estrogen), and improve insulin sensitivity.

- **Strength Training**: Building muscle through resistance exercises can improve metabolic function, boost insulin sensitivity, and support healthy hormone levels.

- **Aerobic Exercise**: Activities like walking, swimming, or cycling can help reduce body fat and lower the risk of estrogen dominance by reducing fat tissue that produces excess estrogen.

3. Detoxification and Reducing Endocrine Disruptors

Endocrine-disrupting chemicals (EDCs) found in plastics, personal care products, and food packaging can mimic estrogen in the body and contribute to estrogen dominance. To support hormone balance, it's important to reduce exposure to these chemicals:

- **Avoid plastic food containers**: Opt for glass or stainless steel when storing food to reduce exposure to harmful chemicals like **BPA**.

- **Choose natural beauty products**: Look for personal care products that are free from parabens and phthalates, both of which can act as endocrine disruptors.

- **Support liver detoxification**: Your liver is responsible for metabolizing and eliminating excess estrogen from the body. Eating foods that support liver health—such as **cruciferous vegetables** (broccoli, cauliflower, Brussels sprouts)—can enhance detoxification and promote hormonal balance.

Conclusion: Taking Control of Your Hormone Health

Estrogen plays a pivotal role in your metabolic and mental health, influencing everything from insulin sensitivity and fat distribution to mood and cognitive function. By understanding how estrogen interacts with other hormones and neurotransmitters, you can take proactive steps to balance your hormones and improve your overall well-being. Through a combination of dietary choices, regular exercise, and reducing exposure to harmful chemicals, you can support your body's natural estrogen balance and take charge of your health.

Chapter 3

PROGESTERONE

THE CALMING HORMONE

PROGESTERONE IS OFTEN CALLED the "calming hormone" because of its profound effects on mood stabilization, sleep, and overall hormonal balance. While estrogen often takes center stage in discussions about female hormones, progesterone is equally important in maintaining equilibrium within the body. From its role in preparing the body for pregnancy to its calming effects on the brain, progesterone is a hormone that influences almost every aspect of a woman's well-being.

In this chapter, we'll explore how progesterone works to promote emotional stability, improve sleep, and maintain hormonal balance. We'll also look at the consequences of low progesterone levels, particularly how they contribute to anxiety, depression, and hormonal imbalances like estrogen dominance. Finally, we'll provide practical, research-backed strategies for naturally boosting progesterone levels through diet, herbs, and stress management techniques.

The Importance of Progesterone for Mood Stabilization, Sleep, and Hormonal Balance

Progesterone is produced primarily by the ovaries after ovulation during the **luteal phase** of the menstrual cycle. This hormone works in concert with estrogen to regulate the reproductive system and prepare the body for a possible pregnancy. However, its effects go far beyond reproduction.

In addition to its role in the menstrual cycle, progesterone exerts a calming effect on the central nervous system, which is why it is often referred to as the body's natural **anxiolytic**—a substance that reduces anxiety. Progesterone is also crucial for promoting restful sleep, regulating other hormones, and keeping estrogen in check, preventing estrogen dominance. Let's take a closer look at how progesterone achieves these effects.

1. Mood Stabilization

One of the most well-known effects of progesterone is its ability to stabilize mood. This is largely due to its interaction with the brain's **GABA (gamma-aminobutyric acid) receptors**, which are responsible for promoting feelings of calm and relaxation. GABA is the brain's primary inhibitory neurotransmitter, meaning it helps reduce neural activity and prevents overstimulation. Progesterone enhances the activity of GABA, creating a sense of tranquility and helping to relieve feelings of anxiety or irritability.

During the luteal phase, when progesterone levels are high, many women experience a sense of calm and emotional balance. However, if progesterone levels are too low, this calming effect is diminished, leading to mood swings, anxiety, and even depression.

2. Sleep Regulation

Progesterone is also essential for promoting restful sleep. Its interaction with GABA not only calms the brain but also prepares the body for deep, restorative sleep. This is why women with balanced progesterone levels often experience better sleep quality during the luteal phase of their menstrual cycle.

However, when progesterone levels drop—such as during perimenopause or in women with **luteal phase defects**—sleep disturbances can become a common issue. Low progesterone is linked to insomnia, restless sleep, and waking up frequently during the night. Many women who suffer from **premenstrual syndrome (PMS)** or perimenopausal symptoms report significant sleep issues, often due to the sharp decline in progesterone that occurs during these times.

3. Hormonal Balance

Progesterone plays a key role in maintaining overall hormonal balance, particularly in relation to estrogen. It helps to "counterbalance" estrogen's effects on the body. While estrogen is essential for many bodily functions, too much of it—particularly when unopposed by sufficient progesterone—can lead to **estrogen dominance**. This hormonal imbalance is linked to a variety of symptoms, including weight gain, mood swings, breast tenderness, and a higher risk of conditions such as fibroids and endometriosis.

Progesterone helps prevent estrogen dominance by regulating the growth-promoting effects of estrogen, particularly on the reproductive organs. It keeps the uterine lining from growing too thick, reducing the risk of conditions like endometrial hyperplasia, which can develop into cancer if left unchecked.

In addition, progesterone has anti-inflammatory effects that help regulate the immune system and maintain a healthy balance between estrogen and other hormones in the body.

How Low Progesterone Leads to Anxiety, Depression, and Hormonal Imbalances

Low progesterone levels can have far-reaching effects on both mental and physical health. When progesterone is deficient, it not only disrupts the menstrual cycle but also causes significant changes in mood and emotional well-being. Here's how:

1. Anxiety and Depression

As mentioned earlier, progesterone enhances the activity of GABA, the brain's natural "calming" neurotransmitter. When progesterone levels are low, GABA activity decreases, leading to increased anxiety, irritability, and a heightened stress response. This is why many women with low progesterone levels experience **anxiety disorders** or **depression**, particularly during the luteal phase of the menstrual cycle, when progesterone should be at its peak.

In women with **premenstrual dysphoric disorder (PMDD)**, a more severe form of PMS, the drop in progesterone before menstruation can lead to severe mood disturbances, including anxiety, depression, and even suicidal thoughts. These emotional changes are directly linked to the hormonal fluctuations of the menstrual cycle and highlight the importance of maintaining balanced progesterone levels for mental health.

2. Estrogen Dominance

Low progesterone is one of the main causes of **estrogen dominance**, a condition in which the body has too much estrogen relative to progesterone. Estrogen dominance can cause a range of symptoms, including:

- **Weight gain**, particularly around the hips and thighs

- **Breast tenderness** and **fibrocystic breasts**

- **Mood swings** and **irritability**

- **Irregular periods** or **heavy bleeding**

- Increased risk of **fibroids**, **endometriosis**, and **breast cancer**

Estrogen dominance often occurs during perimenopause when progesterone levels begin to decline earlier and more rapidly than estrogen levels. It can also be caused by factors such as chronic stress, obesity (fat cells produce estrogen), or exposure to **xenoestrogens**, chemicals in the environment that mimic estrogen.

In addition to these symptoms, estrogen dominance is also linked to a higher risk of **insulin resistance**, a condition in which the body's cells become less responsive to insulin, leading to high blood sugar and an increased risk of type 2 diabetes.

3. Infertility and Miscarriage

Progesterone is critical for supporting pregnancy and maintaining a healthy uterine environment. After ovulation, progesterone prepares the uterine lining (endometrium) for the implantation of a fertilized egg. If progesterone levels are too low, the uterine lining may not be thick enough to support implantation, leading to infertility.

For women who do become pregnant, low progesterone can increase the risk of **miscarriage**. Progesterone is essential during the first trimester of pregnancy to maintain the uterine lining and prevent the body from rejecting the developing embryo. Women with low progesterone levels during early pregnancy may require **progesterone supplementation** to reduce the risk of miscarriage.

Research Highlight: The Link Between Progesterone, GABA, and Relaxation

One of the most fascinating aspects of progesterone's role in the body is its relationship with **GABA**, the brain's primary inhibitory neurotransmitter. GABA is responsible for reducing neural activity, which promotes relaxation and calmness. It acts as a natural tranquilizer, helping to prevent overstimulation in the brain.

Progesterone directly influences GABA receptors, particularly in the areas of the brain responsible for regulating mood and emotional responses. When progesterone levels are sufficient, GABA activity is enhanced, leading to feelings of relaxation, reduced anxiety, and improved emotional resilience.

How Progesterone Boosts GABA Activity

1. **Increased GABA Binding**: Progesterone increases the ability of GABA to bind to its receptors in the brain, amplifying its calming effects. This makes it easier for the brain to "slow down" and prevents the overactivity that often leads to anxiety and stress.

2. **Neurosteroid Effects**: Progesterone is also converted into **allopregnanolone**, a neurosteroid that further enhances GABA activity. Allopregnanolone is a potent modulator of the GABA-A receptor, and its calming effects are similar to those produced by anti-anxiety medications like benzodiazepines. However, unlike pharmaceutical interventions, progesterone's natural effect on GABA is more subtle and supports long-term emotional balance.

The GABA-Progesterone-Anxiety Connection

Research has shown that women with low progesterone levels, particularly during the luteal phase of their cycle, have decreased GABA activity, which is closely linked to the development of **anxiety** and **mood disorders**. A study published in the journal *Neuroscience* found that fluctuations in allopregnanolone (the neurosteroid derived from progesterone) directly correlate with mood changes in women, particularly those with PMS or PMDD.

This research highlights the critical role that progesterone plays in mood regulation and suggests that addressing progesterone deficiency could be an effective strategy for reducing anxiety and improving emotional well-being.

Natural Ways to Boost Progesterone

While hormone replacement therapy (HRT) is often recommended for women with severely low progesterone levels, there are also several natural ways to support healthy progesterone production. By incorporating certain herbs, dietary changes, and stress management techniques, you can help balance your progesterone levels and improve overall hormonal health.

1. Herbal Remedies

Several herbs have been shown to naturally boost progesterone levels by supporting the body's hormonal pathways. These herbs are often referred to as **phyto-progestins** because they mimic the effects of progesterone in the body.

- **Vitex (Chasteberry)**: Vitex is one of the most well-known herbs for promoting progesterone production. It works by stimulating the **pituitary gland** to increase luteinizing hormone (LH) production, which signals the ovaries to produce more progesterone. Vitex is particularly helpful for women with luteal phase defects or irregular cycles.

- **Maca Root**: Maca is an adaptogenic herb that supports overall hormone balance by nourishing the **hypothalamus** and **pituitary glands**, which regulate hormone production. It can help balance progesterone levels and alleviate symptoms of PMS and perimenopause.

- **Red Raspberry Leaf**: Red raspberry leaf is traditionally used to tone the uterus and support reproductive health. It can help regulate the menstrual cycle and support progesterone production, particularly in women who experience heavy periods or irregular cycles.

- **Wild Yam**: Wild yam contains compounds that can be converted into progesterone in the body. While it doesn't contain progesterone itself, wild yam is often used in natural progesterone creams to support hormonal balance.

2. Diet and Nutrition

Certain foods can help boost progesterone production by supporting overall hormonal health and providing the nutrients necessary for hormone synthesis.

- **Magnesium-Rich Foods**: Magnesium is essential for hormone production and regulation. Foods rich in magnesium, such as spinach, pumpkin seeds, almonds, and dark chocolate, can help support healthy progesterone levels.

- **Vitamin B6**: Vitamin B6 plays a crucial role in progesterone production by supporting the body's ability to convert tryptophan into serotonin, which indirectly influences progesterone levels. Foods high in vitamin B6 include chickpeas, bananas, potatoes, and poultry.

- **Zinc**: Zinc is another important nutrient for progesterone production. It helps stimulate the pituitary gland to release follicle-stimulating hormone (FSH), which is necessary for ovulation and progesterone production. Foods high in zinc include oysters, beef, pumpkin seeds, and lentils.

- **Healthy Fats**: Progesterone is synthesized from cholesterol, so consuming healthy fats is essential for hormone production. Focus on including sources of healthy fats, such as avocados, olive oil, fatty fish, and nuts, in your diet.

3. Stress Management

Chronic stress is one of the primary causes of low progesterone levels. When you're under stress, your body produces more **cortisol**, the stress hormone, which competes with progesterone for the same precursor molecules. This process, known as the **pregnenolone steal**, diverts resources away from progesterone production, leading to lower levels of this crucial hormone.

Implementing stress management techniques is essential for maintaining healthy progesterone levels:

- **Mindfulness and Meditation**: Practicing mindfulness and meditation can reduce cortisol levels and improve emotional resilience. Studies have shown that regular meditation helps regulate the **HPA axis** (the body's stress response system), allowing for better hormonal balance.

- **Exercise**: Regular physical activity can help reduce stress, lower cortisol, and support overall hormonal balance. However, it's important to avoid over-exercising, as excessive physical activity can raise cortisol levels and further deplete progesterone.

- **Sleep**: Getting enough high-quality sleep is crucial for hormonal health. Aim for at least 7-9 hours of sleep per night to allow your body to recover and produce adequate progesterone.

Conclusion: Empowering Yourself to Support Healthy Progesterone Levels

Progesterone is a vital hormone that does much more than support reproductive health—it plays a crucial role in emotional well-being, sleep, and overall hormonal balance. When progesterone levels are too low, it can lead to a range of physical and mental health issues, from anxiety and insomnia to estrogen dominance and fertility challenges. By understanding the importance of progesterone and taking proactive steps to support its production, you can improve your hormonal health and enhance your overall well-being.

Whether through herbal remedies, dietary changes, or stress management techniques, there are many ways to naturally boost progesterone levels and achieve a sense of balance and calm. Taking charge of your hormonal health is not only empowering but also essential for maintaining long-term physical and emotional vitality.

Chapter 4

Thyroid Hormones

The Metabolic Regulators

Thyroid hormones, often referred to as the "metabolic regulators," play an essential role in maintaining energy production, metabolism, and overall health. These hormones—**thyroxine (T4)** and **triiodothyronine (T3)**—are produced by the thyroid gland, a small butterfly-shaped gland located at the front of your neck. Though small in size, the thyroid has a powerful influence on nearly every cell and organ in your body. Thyroid hormones regulate metabolism, determine how much energy your body produces, and affect critical functions such as body temperature, heart rate, and even mood.

In this chapter, we'll explore the vital role thyroid hormones play in your overall health, what happens when they become imbalanced, and how these imbalances lead to common conditions like **hypothyroidism** and **hyperthyroidism**. We'll also look at the connection between thyroid hormones and other hormones, including cortisol and estrogen, and how thyroid dysfunction can impact mental health, causing symptoms such as **depression** and **brain fog**. Finally, we'll discuss effective strategies for supporting thyroid function through diet, exercise, and lifestyle adjustments.

The Thyroid's Role in Metabolism, Energy Production, and Overall Health

The thyroid gland produces two primary hormones—T4 and T3—that control the body's **metabolic rate**. Metabolism is the process by which your body converts food into energy. This energy is used for everything from powering your muscles to maintaining your body temperature and supporting brain function. Thyroid hormones regulate how quickly or slowly this process happens, which is why they are often referred to as the body's "thermostat."

1. Thyroxine (T4) and Triiodothyronine (T3)

- **T4 (Thyroxine)**: T4 is the most abundant thyroid hormone produced by the thyroid gland, but it is relatively inactive. Its primary role is to serve as a **prohormone**—a storage form of thyroid hormone that can be converted into T3 when needed.

- **T3 (Triiodothyronine)**: T3 is the active form of thyroid hormone and is responsible for most of the thyroid's effects on the body. T3 is more potent than T4, and it works by entering cells and binding to thyroid hormone receptors. This interaction activates processes that boost metabolism, increase energy production, and regulate cell growth and repair.

Approximately 80% of the thyroid hormone released by the thyroid is T4, which is then converted into T3 in the liver, kidneys, and other tissues. This conversion is critical for maintaining a healthy metabolism.

2. Regulating Energy Production

One of the primary functions of thyroid hormones is to regulate energy production by stimulating the production of **ATP (adenosine triphosphate)**, the molecule that provides energy to cells. T3 increases the number of **mitochondria** (the energy factories of cells) and boosts their activity, allowing them to produce more ATP. This increase in ATP production supports essential bodily functions such as muscle contraction, brain activity, and digestion.

When thyroid hormone levels are normal, your metabolism functions efficiently, allowing you to maintain a healthy weight, feel energetic, and enjoy a sense of well-being. However, when thyroid hormone levels are imbalanced—either too high or too low—it can cause significant disruptions to your energy levels and metabolism.

Hypothyroidism and Hyperthyroidism: How Imbalances Lead to Weight Gain, Fatigue, and Mood Swings

When thyroid hormone levels become imbalanced, they can lead to two primary conditions: **hypothyroidism** (underactive thyroid) and **hyperthyroidism** (overactive thyroid). Both conditions have distinct effects on metabolism, energy levels, and mood.

1. Hypothyroidism: The Underactive Thyroid

Hypothyroidism occurs when the thyroid gland doesn't produce enough T4 and T3 hormones. This condition slows down the body's metabolic processes, resulting in a range of symptoms that can affect everything from weight and energy to mood and cognitive function.

Common Symptoms of Hypothyroidism:

- **Weight Gain**: When thyroid hormone levels are low, the body's metabolic rate decreases, which means fewer calories are burned for energy. As a result, people with hypothyroidism often experience **unexplained weight gain**, even if their diet and activity levels remain the same.

- **Fatigue**: Hypothyroidism can cause **extreme fatigue** and a persistent sense of tiredness. Since T3 is responsible for boosting energy production in cells, low levels of this hormone mean that the body produces less ATP, leaving you feeling sluggish and lacking in energy.

- **Cold Sensitivity**: People with hypothyroidism often feel cold, even in warm environments, because their body produces less heat due to a slower metabolism.

- **Mood Changes**: Hypothyroidism can also affect mood, causing feelings of **depression**, **anxiety**, and **irritability**. The drop in thyroid hormone levels leads to lower levels of neurotransmitters like **serotonin** and **dopamine**, which are essential for regulating mood.

- **Cognitive Difficulties**: Many people with hypothyroidism experience **brain fog**, memory problems, and difficulty concentrating. These cognitive symptoms occur because thyroid hormones are critical for maintaining healthy brain function.

Causes of Hypothyroidism:

- **Hashimoto's Thyroiditis**: The most common cause of hypothyroidism is an autoimmune disorder called Hashimoto's thyroiditis. In this condition, the immune system mistakenly attacks the thyroid gland, causing inflammation and reducing its ability to produce hormones.

- **Iodine Deficiency**: Iodine is a key component of thyroid hormones, and a deficiency in this mineral can impair thyroid function. While iodine deficiency is rare in many developed countries due to the use of iodized salt, it remains a concern in some parts of the world.

2. Hyperthyroidism: The Overactive Thyroid

Hyperthyroidism occurs when the thyroid gland produces too much T4 and T3. This condition speeds up the body's metabolic processes, leading to a range of symptoms that are often the opposite of hypothyroidism.

Common Symptoms of Hyperthyroidism:

- **Weight Loss**: People with hyperthyroidism often experience **unintentional weight loss** because their body's metabolism is in overdrive. Despite eating more, their body burns through calories quickly, leading to weight loss.

- **Increased Heart Rate and Palpitations**: Hyperthyroidism can cause an increased heart rate, **palpitations**, and a feeling of being constantly "on edge." This is due to the heightened activity of the body's **sympathetic nervous system**.

- **Nervousness and Irritability**: The excess production of thyroid hormones can lead to **nervousness**, **anxiety**, and **irritability**, as the body is in a constant state of overstimulation.

- **Heat Intolerance**: People with hyperthyroidism often feel hot and sweaty, even in cooler environments. This is because their increased metabolic rate generates more body heat.

- **Fatigue**: While hyperthyroidism can cause a burst of energy in the short term, over time, it leads to **fatigue** and **muscle weakness** as the body becomes exhausted from being in a constant state of overdrive.

Causes of Hyperthyroidism:

- **Graves' Disease**: The most common cause of hyperthyroidism is an autoimmune disorder called **Graves' disease**. In this condition, the immune system produces antibodies that stimulate the thyroid gland to produce too much hormone.

- **Thyroid Nodules**: Hyperthyroidism can also be caused by **thyroid nodules**, which are small growths in the thyroid gland that produce excess thyroid hormone.

The Connection Between Thyroid Hormones (T3, T4) and Other Hormones Like Cortisol and Estrogen

Thyroid hormones don't act in isolation—they interact with other hormones in the body, creating a complex hormonal balance that affects overall health. The most notable interactions are between thyroid hormones, **cortisol** (the stress hormone), and **estrogen**.

1. Thyroid Hormones and Cortisol

Cortisol, produced by the adrenal glands, is the body's primary stress hormone. It plays a key role in regulating the body's stress response, metabolism, and immune function. However, chronic stress and elevated cortisol levels can disrupt thyroid function.

- **Cortisol's Impact on Thyroid Function**: Chronic stress can lead to **adrenal fatigue**, which in turn affects thyroid hormone production. High levels of cortisol interfere with the conversion of T4 into T3, reducing the availability of active thyroid hormone in the body. This can lead to symptoms of hypothyroidism, even if the thyroid gland is functioning normally.

- **The Thyroid-Adrenal Axis**: The thyroid and adrenal glands work closely together in what is known as the **thyroid-adrenal axis**. When the body is under chronic stress, the adrenal glands prioritize the production of cortisol over other hormones, leading to a downregulation of thyroid hormone production. This interplay between cortisol and thyroid hormones highlights the importance of stress management in maintaining thyroid health.

2. Thyroid Hormones and Estrogen

Estrogen, the primary female sex hormone, also has a significant influence on thyroid function. The relationship between estrogen and thyroid hormones is particularly important for women, as fluctuations in estrogen levels can affect thyroid hormone levels.

- **Estrogen's Impact on Thyroid Binding Globulin (TBG)**: Estrogen increases the production of **thyroid binding globulin (TBG),** a protein that binds to thyroid hormones in the blood. When more TBG is present, less free T4 and T3 are available for use by the body's cells. This is why some women experience symptoms of hypothyroidism during periods of high estrogen levels, such as pregnancy or when using hormone replacement therapy (HRT).

- **Thyroid Dysfunction and Menstrual Irregularities**: Thyroid hormone imbalances can also affect estrogen levels, leading to **menstrual irregularities**. For example, women with hypothyroidism often experience heavy or irregular periods due to disrupted estrogen metabolism. Conversely, hyperthyroidism can cause lighter or absent periods.

Research Highlight: The Connection Between Thyroid Health and Mental Health (Depression, Brain Fog)

The thyroid's influence on mental health is profound. Research has shown that thyroid hormone imbalances are closely linked to mood disorders such as **depression** and **anxiety**, as well as cognitive issues like **brain fog** and memory problems.

1. Depression and Hypothyroidism

People with hypothyroidism are more likely to experience **depression** and **low mood** due to the reduced production of neurotransmitters like serotonin and dopamine, which are critical for maintaining emotional stability. A study published in the *Journal of Clinical Psychiatry* found that people with untreated hypothyroidism are significantly more likely to experience depressive symptoms compared to those with normal thyroid function.

Hypothyroidism also slows down cognitive processes, leading to feelings of **mental sluggishness** and difficulty concentrating. This phenomenon, often referred to as **brain fog**, is common in people with thyroid dysfunction and can severely impact daily functioning and quality of life.

2. Anxiety and Hyperthyroidism

On the other hand, hyperthyroidism can cause heightened levels of **anxiety** and **nervousness** due to the overstimulation of the nervous system. The excess production of thyroid hormones leads to increased activity in the brain's stress pathways, which can cause a constant state of mental hyperactivity and emotional instability.

Strategies to Support Thyroid Function

Maintaining optimal thyroid health is essential for overall well-being. While some thyroid conditions may require medical treatment, there are several dietary and lifestyle strategies that can support healthy thyroid function.

1. Selenium

Selenium is a trace mineral that plays a key role in the conversion of T4 into T3, the active form of thyroid hormone. Selenium also has powerful antioxidant properties that protect the thyroid gland from oxidative stress and inflammation.

- **Food Sources of Selenium**: Brazil nuts are one of the best dietary sources of selenium. Just one or two Brazil nuts per day can provide the recommended daily intake of selenium.

Other good sources include tuna, eggs, and sunflower seeds.

2. Iodine

Iodine is an essential component of thyroid hormones, as both T4 and T3 contain iodine atoms. Without adequate iodine intake, the thyroid cannot produce sufficient thyroid hormones, leading to hypothyroidism.

- **Food Sources of Iodine**: Seaweed, such as kelp, is one of the richest sources of iodine. Iodized salt, fish, and dairy products also provide significant amounts of iodine.

3. Dietary Changes

Eating a diet that supports thyroid health is critical for maintaining balanced hormone levels. Focus on nutrient-rich foods that provide the vitamins and minerals necessary for thyroid function.

- **Avoid Goitrogens**: Certain foods, known as **goitrogens**, can interfere with thyroid hormone production. These include cruciferous vegetables like broccoli, cauliflower, and cabbage. While these foods are healthy in moderation, people with hypothyroidism should avoid consuming large quantities of raw goitrogenic vegetables.

- **Increase Antioxidants**: Antioxidant-rich foods, such as berries, leafy greens, and colorful vegetables, help protect the thyroid from oxidative stress.

4. Regular Exercise

Physical activity boosts metabolism and supports thyroid health. Exercise stimulates the production of thyroid hormones and increases the body's sensitivity to T3, enhancing energy production and overall metabolic function.

- **Moderate-Intensity Exercise**: Activities such as walking, swimming, or cycling can help improve thyroid function without overstressing the body. High-intensity exercise may exacerbate symptoms in people with hyperthyroidism, so it's important to find a balance that works for your body.

5. Stress Management

Chronic stress can have a detrimental effect on thyroid health due to its impact on cortisol levels. Practicing stress management techniques such as meditation, deep breathing, and yoga can help lower cortisol levels and improve thyroid function.

Conclusion: Taking Control of Your Thyroid Health

The thyroid gland is a powerful regulator of metabolism, energy production, and mental well-being. Understanding how thyroid hormones work—and how imbalances can affect your health—is essential for maintaining optimal thyroid function. By supporting your thyroid with proper nutrition, regular exercise, stress management, and targeted supplements like selenium and iodine, you can improve your overall health and take control of your metabolism and energy levels.

Empowering yourself with the knowledge and tools to support thyroid health can help you avoid the common pitfalls of thyroid imbalances, such as weight gain, fatigue, and mood swings. Whether you're managing a diagnosed thyroid condition or simply looking to optimize your thyroid function, these strategies can help you live a healthier, more vibrant life.

PART II

Hormones and Mental Health

Chapter 5

DEPRESSION, ANXIETY, AND HORMONAL IMBALANCE

HORMONES AND NEUROTRANSMITTERS INTERACT in complex ways, and imbalances in hormones such as **estrogen**, **cortisol**, **progesterone**, and **thyroid hormones** can have profound effects on the brain's chemistry. Specifically, these hormonal shifts influence **serotonin** and **dopamine**, two key neurotransmitters that regulate mood, emotions, and mental clarity. When hormones are imbalanced, the delicate relationship between hormones and neurotransmitters can be disrupted, leading to mood disorders such as **depression**, **anxiety**, and **irritability**.

This section delves into the intricate relationship between hormone imbalances and brain health, how hormonal changes during the menstrual cycle, pregnancy, and menopause can contribute to mood disorders, and provides actionable strategies—both natural and medical—for treating hormone-related depression and anxiety.

The Role of Neurotransmitters: Serotonin and Dopamine

Before diving into how hormone imbalances affect mood, let's first understand the role of the two main neurotransmitters involved in mood regulation: **serotonin** and **dopamine**.

- **Serotonin** is often called the "feel-good" neurotransmitter. It is responsible for promoting feelings of happiness, emotional stability, and overall well-being. Serotonin helps regulate mood, sleep, appetite, and cognitive function. Low serotonin levels are closely linked to depression, anxiety, and insomnia.

- **Dopamine** is often referred to as the "reward" neurotransmitter. It plays a key role in motivation, pleasure, and focus. When dopamine levels are balanced, you feel motivated, focused, and emotionally stable. Imbalances in dopamine can lead to low motivation, depression, and even addictive behaviors.

Both serotonin and dopamine levels are highly sensitive to changes in hormone levels. That's why many women experience mood changes during different phases of their menstrual cycle, pregnancy, or menopause—times when hormone levels fluctuate dramatically.

Estrogen and Neurotransmitters: A Powerful Connection

Estrogen is one of the most important hormones when it comes to regulating neurotransmitters like serotonin and dopamine. Estrogen increases the production of serotonin and enhances the sensitivity

DEPRESSION, ANXIETY, AND HORMONAL IMBALANCE

of serotonin receptors in the brain. This means that when estrogen levels are balanced, serotonin can do its job effectively, promoting stable mood and emotional well-being.

1. Estrogen and Serotonin Production

Estrogen directly affects the enzyme **tryptophan hydroxylase**, which is responsible for converting the amino acid **tryptophan** into serotonin in the brain. Higher estrogen levels lead to increased serotonin production, which helps explain why many women feel more emotionally stable and happy during the **follicular phase** of their menstrual cycle, when estrogen levels are at their peak.

Conversely, when estrogen levels drop—such as during **premenstrual syndrome (PMS)** or **menopause**—serotonin production declines. This reduction in serotonin is one of the main reasons why many women experience mood swings, depression, and irritability before their periods or during menopause.

2. Estrogen and Dopamine

Estrogen also affects **dopamine** levels by increasing dopamine receptor density in the brain's reward centers. This enhances the brain's ability to feel pleasure, motivation, and focus. Women with balanced estrogen levels tend to have better cognitive function, greater motivation, and a more positive outlook. However, when estrogen levels fall—such as during perimenopause or postpartum—dopamine levels drop as well, leading to **anhedonia** (the inability to feel pleasure), low motivation, and even **depression**.

3. Estrogen Deficiency and Mood Disorders

Estrogen deficiency, particularly during menopause, can lead to significant mood disturbances. Studies show that women going through menopause are more likely to experience **depression**, **anxiety**, and **cognitive decline**. This is because the sudden drop in estrogen affects serotonin and dopamine production, leaving the brain less equipped to manage mood and emotional well-being.

In fact, research published in the *Journal of Women's Health* has shown that women are two to three times more likely to experience **major depressive disorder** during menopause compared to women in their reproductive years. Hormone replacement therapy (HRT), particularly **bioidentical hormone replacement therapy (BHRT)**, has been shown to help mitigate these mood disturbances by restoring estrogen levels and promoting healthy neurotransmitter function.

Cortisol: The Stress Hormone's Impact on Mood

Cortisol is the body's primary stress hormone, produced by the adrenal glands in response to stress. While cortisol is essential for managing short-term stress, chronically elevated cortisol levels can wreak havoc on mood and mental well-being.

1. Cortisol and Serotonin

Cortisol interacts with serotonin in complex ways. Under chronic stress, elevated cortisol levels can reduce **serotonin receptor sensitivity**, making it harder for serotonin to bind to its receptors in the brain. This reduces serotonin's effectiveness, leading to feelings of sadness, anxiety, and depression.

Additionally, high cortisol levels interfere with the production of **serotonin precursors**, further reducing serotonin availability. This is one of the reasons why chronic stress is a major risk factor for developing **depression** and **anxiety disorders**.

2. Cortisol and Dopamine

Elevated cortisol levels can also suppress dopamine production. Since dopamine is responsible for motivation, pleasure, and reward, people with high cortisol levels often feel **burnt out**, lack motivation, and may experience **anhedonia**. This is why chronic stress can lead to **adrenal fatigue**, a condition characterized by low energy, low mood, and a lack of pleasure in everyday activities.

3. Chronic Stress and Mental Health

Chronic stress and the accompanying high cortisol levels not only disrupt neurotransmitter function but also affect the **hippocampus**, the part of the brain responsible for memory and learning. Over time, chronic stress can lead to **brain fog**, poor concentration, and memory issues.

The connection between cortisol and mental health is particularly relevant for women in today's fast-paced society, where chronic stress is becoming increasingly common. Stress management techniques such as **mindfulness**, **meditation**, and **deep breathing** are effective ways to reduce cortisol levels and protect mental health.

Progesterone: The Calming Hormone

While estrogen gets much of the attention, **progesterone** is equally important for mental and emotional health. Progesterone is often called the "calming hormone" because of its interaction with **GABA (gamma-aminobutyric acid)**, the brain's primary inhibitory neurotransmitter.

1. Progesterone and GABA

GABA is responsible for promoting relaxation, reducing anxiety, and calming the brain. Progesterone increases GABA's activity by binding to **GABA receptors**, enhancing its calming effects. This is why many women feel a sense of calm and emotional stability during the **luteal phase** of their menstrual cycle, when progesterone levels are high.

However, when progesterone levels drop—such as during **premenstrual syndrome (PMS)** or **perimenopause**—GABA activity is reduced, leading to increased anxiety, irritability, and **mood swings**.

2. Progesterone Deficiency and Anxiety

Progesterone deficiency can lead to **anxiety**, **restlessness**, and **insomnia**. This is especially true for women with **premenstrual dysphoric disorder (PMDD)**, a more severe form of PMS characterized by extreme mood swings, anxiety, and depression. Women with PMDD often experience a significant drop in progesterone during the luteal phase, which disrupts GABA activity and triggers mood disorders.

Progesterone therapy, particularly **bioidentical progesterone**, has been shown to help reduce anxiety and improve mood in women with progesterone deficiency by restoring GABA activity in the brain.

Thyroid Hormones: Essential for Brain and Mood Health

Thyroid hormones—**T3 (triiodothyronine)** and **T4 (thyroxine)**—regulate metabolism, energy production, and brain function. Imbalances in thyroid hormones, such as **hypothyroidism** (underactive thyroid) or **hyperthyroidism** (overactive thyroid), can have significant effects on mood, energy levels, and cognitive function.

1. Hypothyroidism and Depression

Hypothyroidism, characterized by low thyroid hormone levels, is closely linked to **depression**. The thyroid hormones T3 and T4 are essential for serotonin production and neurotransmitter regulation. When thyroid hormone levels are low, serotonin production decreases, leading to low mood, fatigue, and cognitive difficulties like **brain fog** and **memory problems**.

Studies have shown that people with untreated hypothyroidism are significantly more likely to experience depression. Many patients with **subclinical hypothyroidism** (mildly low thyroid function) report symptoms of depression, even if their thyroid hormone levels are within the normal range.

2. Hyperthyroidism and Anxiety

On the other hand, **hyperthyroidism**—a condition in which the thyroid produces too much hormone—can lead to **anxiety**, **restlessness**, and **irritability**. The excess thyroid hormone overstimulates the nervous system, leading to a constant state of heightened arousal and anxiety. People with hyperthyroidism often experience **insomnia**, **nervousness**, and difficulty relaxing due to the overstimulation of neurotransmitter pathways.

3. Thyroid Hormones and Brain Health

Thyroid hormones are also critical for brain development and cognitive function. In fact, hypothyroidism has been linked to **cognitive decline** and an increased risk of **dementia**. Maintaining balanced thyroid hormone levels is essential for protecting brain health and ensuring optimal cognitive performance.

Hormonal Changes and Mood Disorders: The Menstrual Cycle, Pregnancy, and Menopause

Hormonal fluctuations throughout a woman's life—during the menstrual cycle, pregnancy, and menopause—can have significant effects on mood and mental well-being.

1. The Menstrual Cycle and Mood

The menstrual cycle involves fluctuating levels of estrogen, progesterone, and other hormones that can directly impact mood. Many women experience **premenstrual syndrome (PMS)** in the days leading up to their period, characterized by mood swings, irritability, and depression. These symptoms are often due to the sharp drop in estrogen and progesterone that occurs during the luteal phase.

In more severe cases, women may experience **premenstrual dysphoric disorder (PMDD)**, a condition that causes extreme mood disturbances, including severe anxiety and depression. PMDD is thought to be caused by abnormal sensitivity to normal hormone fluctuations, particularly progesterone.

2. Pregnancy and Postpartum Depression

Pregnancy is associated with dramatic hormonal changes that can affect mental health. While many women experience feelings of joy and excitement during pregnancy, others may struggle with **prenatal depression** or **anxiety**. After childbirth, estrogen and progesterone levels drop sharply, which can trigger **postpartum depression**. This condition affects up to 15% of new mothers and is characterized by severe depression, anxiety, and difficulty bonding with the baby.

3. Menopause and Mood Disorders

Menopause is a time of significant hormonal change, particularly a decline in estrogen and progesterone levels. These hormonal shifts can lead to a range of **menopausal symptoms**, including **mood swings**, **depression**, and **anxiety**. Many women report feeling emotionally unstable or "out of control" as they transition through menopause due to the fluctuating hormone levels and their effects on neurotransmitter production.

Research Highlight: The Impact of Hormonal Fluctuations on Brain Health and Mental Well-Being

The connection between hormones and mental health is well-documented. Research has shown that hormonal fluctuations, whether due to the menstrual cycle, pregnancy, or menopause, can significantly impact **brain health** and **mental well-being**.

A study published in the *Journal of Clinical Endocrinology & Metabolism* found that women are twice as likely as men to experience **mood disorders**, largely due to the effects of hormonal fluctuations on neurotransmitter function. The study highlighted the critical role that estrogen, progesterone, cortisol, and thyroid hormones play in regulating mood, emotions, and cognitive function.

Additionally, research has shown that hormone-related mood disorders, such as **premenstrual dysphoric disorder (PMDD)** and **postpartum depression**, are associated with abnormalities in neurotransmitter sensitivity, particularly serotonin and dopamine.

Natural and Medical Treatments for Hormone-related Depression and Anxiety

Treating hormone-related mood disorders requires a holistic approach that addresses both the underlying hormonal imbalances and the resulting neurotransmitter dysfunction. Fortunately, there are a range of natural and medical treatments that can help restore balance and improve mental well-being.

1. Bioidentical Hormone Replacement Therapy (BHRT)

Bioidentical hormone replacement therapy (BHRT) is a natural form of hormone therapy that uses hormones identical to those produced by the body. BHRT is often recommended for women going through menopause or for those with hormonal deficiencies, such as low estrogen or progesterone levels. By restoring hormone levels, BHRT can help alleviate mood disorders, improve energy levels, and enhance overall well-being.

2. Diet and Nutrition

Diet plays a critical role in balancing hormones and supporting neurotransmitter production. Certain nutrients, such as **omega-3 fatty acids**, **magnesium**, and **B vitamins**, are essential for neurotransmitter function and can help improve mood.

- **Omega-3 Fatty Acids**: Found in fish like salmon and mackerel, omega-3s support serotonin function and reduce inflammation, helping to stabilize mood.

- **Magnesium**: This mineral supports GABA activity and helps reduce anxiety. Foods rich in magnesium include spinach, almonds, and dark chocolate.

- **B Vitamins**: B vitamins, particularly **B6** and **B12**, are essential for neurotransmitter production. Foods rich in B vitamins include eggs, poultry, and leafy greens.

3. Stress Management

Managing stress is crucial for maintaining hormonal balance and protecting mental health. Techniques such as **meditation**, **yoga**, and **deep breathing** can help reduce cortisol levels and improve emotional well-being. Regular exercise, particularly **aerobic exercise**, has been shown to boost serotonin and dopamine levels, enhancing mood and reducing symptoms of depression and anxiety.

4. Cognitive Behavioral Therapy (CBT)

Cognitive behavioral therapy (CBT) is a proven psychological treatment for depression and anxiety. CBT helps individuals identify and challenge negative thought patterns that contribute to mood disorders. When combined with hormone therapy or lifestyle changes, CBT can be an effective tool for improving mental well-being.

Conclusion: Taking Control of Your Hormonal and Mental Health

Hormonal imbalances have a significant impact on neurotransmitter function, mood, and mental well-being. Whether you're dealing with fluctuations in estrogen, cortisol, progesterone, or thyroid hormones, understanding the connection between hormones and neurotransmitters can empower you to take action to balance your hormones and improve your mental health.

By incorporating natural treatments such as diet, stress management, and lifestyle changes, along with medical interventions like BHRT, you can restore balance to your hormones and neurotransmitters, reduce symptoms of depression and anxiety, and enjoy a greater sense of emotional well-being.

Chapter 6

THE GUT-HORMONE-MIND CONNECTION

The health of your gut plays a crucial role in regulating hormones and maintaining mental well-being. As emerging research continues to uncover the intricate relationship between the **gut microbiome** and hormone regulation, it is becoming increasingly clear that gut health is essential not just for digestion, but for balancing hormones like **estrogen**, **cortisol**, and **thyroid hormones**. The gut is central to overall health, and its influence extends to the brain through what is known as the **gut-brain axis**. Understanding how the gut microbiome influences hormone levels, mood, and mental clarity can empower you to take action and improve your health from the inside out.

In this chapter, we will explore the latest research on the gut-hormone connection, how imbalances in gut health can affect key hormones, and what strategies you can adopt to optimize your gut for better hormonal balance. We will also discuss the impact of gut health on mental clarity, mood regulation, and how to nourish your gut microbiome with practical dietary and lifestyle changes.

The Emerging Science Behind the Gut Microbiome's Role in Hormone Regulation

Your gut contains trillions of microorganisms, including bacteria, fungi, viruses, and other microbes, collectively known as the **gut microbiome**. These microbes play an essential role in digesting food, absorbing nutrients, and maintaining a healthy immune system. However, their influence goes far beyond digestion.

The gut microbiome is now understood to be a key player in hormone regulation, acting as a central hub for hormone metabolism and synthesis. Hormones such as estrogen, cortisol, and thyroid hormones are all influenced by the state of your gut, and any imbalance in your gut microbiome can lead to disruptions in hormone levels.

1. The Gut and Estrogen Metabolism

One of the most important roles of the gut microbiome is its involvement in **estrogen metabolism**. A group of bacteria in the gut, known as the **estrobolome**, is responsible for metabolizing and regulating estrogen levels. These bacteria produce enzymes that help break down estrogen, ensuring it is properly metabolized and excreted from the body.

When the gut microbiome is healthy, estrogen metabolism runs smoothly. However, when gut health is compromised—due to poor diet, antibiotics, or stress—the gut microbiome can become imbalanced, leading to **estrogen dominance**. Estrogen dominance occurs when the body is unable to properly metabolize and eliminate excess estrogen, resulting in symptoms such as weight gain, mood swings, PMS, and an increased risk of estrogen-dependent cancers.

- **Gut Dysbiosis and Estrogen Dominance**: **Gut dysbiosis**, a condition where the balance of good and bad bacteria in the gut is disrupted, can impair estrogen metabolism. Research shows that an imbalanced gut microbiome can lead to the reabsorption of estrogen back into the bloodstream, causing an excess of circulating estrogen. This can contribute to hormonal imbalances such as **premenstrual syndrome (PMS), polycystic ovary syndrome (PCOS),** and **endometriosis**.

A study published in *The Journal of Clinical Endocrinology & Metabolism* found that women with gut dysbiosis were significantly more likely to experience symptoms of estrogen dominance, including bloating, fatigue, and breast tenderness. The study highlighted the importance of maintaining a healthy gut microbiome to support proper estrogen metabolism.

2. The Gut and Cortisol Regulation

The gut microbiome also plays a role in regulating **cortisol**, the body's primary stress hormone. Cortisol is produced by the adrenal glands in response to stress and is essential for managing the body's stress response, immune function, and energy levels. However, chronic stress and poor gut health can lead to elevated cortisol levels, which can disrupt the balance of other hormones.

- **The Gut-Stress Axis**: The **gut-stress axis** is a bidirectional communication pathway between the gut microbiome and the **hypothalamic-pituitary-adrenal (HPA) axis**, which controls cortisol production. When the gut microbiome is healthy, it helps regulate cortisol production by reducing inflammation and promoting resilience to stress. However, when the gut is imbalanced, it can trigger a heightened stress response, leading to increased cortisol production.

A **2017 study published in** *Psychoneuroendocrinology* found that individuals with gut dysbiosis had elevated cortisol levels and were more likely to experience chronic stress, anxiety, and depression. The study also found that improving gut health through diet and probiotics reduced cortisol levels and improved stress resilience.

3. The Gut and Thyroid Function

Thyroid hormones—**T3 (triiodothyronine)** and **T4 (thyroxine)**—are responsible for regulating metabolism, energy production, and overall health. The gut microbiome plays a crucial role in supporting thyroid function by influencing nutrient absorption, reducing inflammation, and regulating the immune system.

- **Gut Health and Thyroid Hormones**: A healthy gut is essential for the absorption of key nutrients like **iodine**, **selenium**, and **zinc**, which are necessary for thyroid hormone production. Gut dysbiosis can impair the absorption of these nutrients, leading to thyroid dysfunction, particularly **hypothyroidism** (underactive thyroid).

- **Autoimmune Thyroid Disorders**: The gut microbiome also plays a role in modulating the immune system, and gut dysbiosis has been linked to autoimmune thyroid disorders such as **Hashimoto's thyroiditis**, a condition in which the immune system attacks the thyroid gland, leading to hypothyroidism.

A **2019 study published in** *Thyroid Research* found that individuals with autoimmune thyroid disorders had significantly lower microbial diversity in their gut compared to healthy individuals. The researchers concluded that improving gut health could help reduce inflammation and support better thyroid function.

Research Highlight: The Link Between Gut Health, Mood, and Mental Clarity (The Gut-Brain Axis)

The gut is often referred to as the **"second brain"** because of its direct connection to the central nervous system through the **vagus nerve** and its production of neurotransmitters like **serotonin**, **dopamine**, and **GABA**. This connection between the gut and the brain is known as the **gut-brain axis**, and it plays a significant role in regulating mood, cognition, and mental clarity.

1. The Gut Microbiome's Role in Neurotransmitter Production

Approximately **90% of the body's serotonin**—the neurotransmitter responsible for mood regulation, happiness, and emotional stability—is produced in the gut. The gut microbiome influences the production and availability of serotonin, as well as other neurotransmitters like dopamine and GABA, which are critical for mental clarity and emotional well-being.

When the gut microbiome is balanced, it supports optimal neurotransmitter production, promoting positive mood and mental clarity. However, an imbalanced gut can disrupt neurotransmitter production, leading to symptoms of **depression, anxiety,** and **brain fog**.

- **Gut Dysbiosis and Mental Health**: Research has shown that individuals with gut dysbiosis are more likely to experience mood disorders such as anxiety and depression. A **2020 study published in *Nature Microbiology*** found that people with lower gut microbial diversity had significantly higher rates of depression and anxiety. The study also found that restoring gut health through the use of probiotics and prebiotics improved mood and mental clarity in the participants.

2. The Gut-Brain Axis and Inflammation

The gut microbiome plays a key role in regulating inflammation, which can directly affect brain health. Chronic inflammation, often caused by poor gut health, has been linked to mood disorders and cognitive decline. The gut microbiome helps modulate the immune response and reduce inflammation, protecting the brain from inflammatory damage.

A **2018 study published in *Frontiers in Psychiatry*** found that individuals with major depressive disorder had elevated levels of inflammatory markers and reduced gut microbial diversity. The study concluded that improving gut health through dietary interventions reduced inflammation and improved symptoms of depression.

Strategies for Optimizing Gut Health for Better Hormone Balance

Now that we understand how critical the gut microbiome is for regulating hormones and mental health, let's explore some practical strategies for improving gut health and achieving better hormonal balance.

1. Increase Fiber Intake

Dietary fiber is essential for feeding the beneficial bacteria in the gut, known as **prebiotics**. Fiber helps maintain a healthy balance of gut bacteria, promotes regular digestion, and supports the elimination of excess hormones like estrogen.

- **Sources of Fiber**: Include fiber-rich foods in your diet such as leafy greens, legumes, whole grains, and fruits like apples and pears. Aim for at least **25-30 grams of fiber** per day to support gut health and hormone metabolism.

A **2019 study published in *Nutrients*** found that women who consumed a high-fiber diet had lower levels of circulating estrogen and reduced risk of developing estrogen-dependent conditions such as breast cancer and endometriosis.

2. Incorporate Probiotics and Fermented Foods

Probiotics are live beneficial bacteria that help restore balance to the gut microbiome. Consuming probiotic-rich foods can improve gut health, enhance hormone metabolism, and reduce inflammation.

- **Sources of Probiotics**: Incorporate fermented foods such as **yogurt, kefir, sauerkraut, kimchi,** and **kombucha** into your diet. These foods provide beneficial bacteria that support gut health and promote a balanced microbiome.

A **2017 study published in** *The American Journal of Clinical Nutrition* found that women who regularly consumed fermented foods had improved gut microbial diversity, reduced symptoms of depression, and better hormonal balance.

3. Include Prebiotics in Your Diet

Prebiotics are non-digestible fibers that feed the good bacteria in your gut, helping them grow and thrive. By promoting the growth of beneficial bacteria, prebiotics support hormone metabolism and neurotransmitter production.

- **Sources of Prebiotics**: Prebiotic-rich foods include garlic, onions, leeks, **asparagus, bananas, chicory root,** and **dandelion greens**. Incorporating these foods into your diet helps nourish the beneficial bacteria in your gut and promotes a balanced microbiome, which in turn supports hormone regulation.

A **2015 study published in** *Frontiers in Endocrinology* found that women who consumed a diet rich in prebiotics had improved gut health, lower levels of cortisol, and better overall hormone balance. The study also found that prebiotic supplementation improved mood and reduced symptoms of anxiety in participants.

4. Reduce Inflammatory Foods

Certain foods can disrupt gut health by promoting inflammation and contributing to gut dysbiosis. These foods include **refined sugars**, **processed foods**, **trans fats**, and **artificial additives**. Inflammation caused by poor dietary choices can disrupt hormone regulation, leading to issues like estrogen dominance, thyroid dysfunction, and elevated cortisol levels.

- **Avoid Processed Foods**: Processed and ultra-processed foods, which are often high in sugar, unhealthy fats, and artificial preservatives, can harm the gut microbiome by feeding harmful bacteria and promoting inflammation. Limiting these foods is critical for maintaining gut and hormone health.

- **Choose Anti-inflammatory Foods**: Focus on anti-inflammatory foods such as **fatty fish** (rich in omega-3 fatty acids), **berries**, **green leafy vegetables**, and **nuts**. Omega-3 fatty acids, in particular, have been shown to support both gut and brain health by reducing inflammation and promoting the growth of beneficial gut bacteria.

A **2019 study in *The Journal of Nutrition*** showed that individuals who followed an anti-inflammatory diet experienced significant improvements in gut microbial diversity, reductions in inflammatory markers, and improvements in hormone regulation, particularly in estrogen metabolism and cortisol balance.

5. Manage Stress to Protect Gut Health

As discussed earlier, chronic stress can disrupt gut health by increasing cortisol levels, which in turn can lead to gut dysbiosis and hormone imbalances. Managing stress is essential for maintaining a healthy gut-brain-hormone connection.

- **Mindfulness and Meditation**: Practicing mindfulness, meditation, or **deep breathing exercises** can help reduce cortisol levels and improve gut health. Stress management techniques have been shown to enhance gut microbial diversity, lower inflammation, and support better hormone balance.

- **Exercise**: Regular physical activity can also improve gut health by promoting the growth of beneficial bacteria and supporting healthy digestion. Exercise reduces cortisol levels and enhances serotonin and dopamine production, which are essential for mental clarity and emotional well-being.

A **2020 study published in** *Psychosomatic Medicine* found that individuals who engaged in regular exercise had a more diverse gut microbiome, lower cortisol levels, and improved hormone balance. The study emphasized that moderate-intensity exercise, such as walking, cycling, or yoga, was particularly effective for improving gut and hormone health.

The Gut-Hormone Connection: A Path to Improved Health and Well-Being

The relationship between the gut, hormones, and the brain is one of the most exciting areas of emerging research in the field of health and wellness. The **gut-hormone-mind connection** highlights the importance of gut health not only for digestion but also for maintaining balanced hormones, stable mood, and mental clarity.

By optimizing your gut health through dietary changes, stress management, and the inclusion of probiotics and prebiotics, you can take control of your hormonal health and improve your overall well-being. The strategies outlined in this chapter—such as increasing fiber intake, consuming fermented foods, and reducing inflammatory foods—are powerful tools for promoting a balanced gut microbiome that supports the regulation of hormones like estrogen, cortisol, and thyroid hormones.

By nourishing your gut, you are actively supporting the balance of hormones that are essential for your physical, mental, and emotional health. Whether you're dealing with hormonal imbalances, stress-related gut issues, or mood disorders, understanding the gut-hormone connection empowers you to take proactive steps toward better health from the inside out.

Conclusion: Taking Control of Your Gut, Hormones, and Mind

As the science behind the gut-hormone-mind connection continues to evolve, it becomes increasingly clear that gut health is a foundational pillar of hormonal balance and mental well-being. The gut microbiome's role in regulating estrogen, cortisol, thyroid hormones, and neurotransmitters like serotonin and dopamine means that a healthy gut is essential for emotional stability, mental clarity, and overall vitality.

By taking charge of your gut health through evidence-based strategies, you can enhance your hormone regulation, reduce symptoms of mood disorders like anxiety and depression, and promote a state of balance and well-being. The key is to recognize the power of your gut and to adopt daily habits that support its health, from nourishing your microbiome with prebiotics and probiotics to managing stress effectively.

Whether you're striving to improve your mood, balance your hormones, or optimize your overall health, focusing on your gut health is one of the most impactful steps you can take. By supporting the gut-brain axis and the gut-hormone connection, you are giving yourself the tools to live a healthier, more balanced life—physically, mentally, and emotionally.

Part III

Food, Hormones, and the Modern Food Industry

Chapter 7

THE FOOD WE EAT AND ITS IMPACT ON HORMONAL HEALTH

WHAT WE EAT IS a powerful factor in determining how well our body's hormones function. The food we choose can either support healthy hormone production and balance or lead to disruptions in key systems like metabolism, reproductive health, and mood regulation. Hormones like **insulin, estrogen, progesterone**, and **thyroid hormones** play central roles in keeping our bodies in sync, and their function is heavily influenced by the nutrients we consume. In this chapter, we'll explore how macronutrients (proteins, carbohydrates, and fats) contribute to hormone production, the harmful effects of sugar, refined carbohydrates, and unhealthy fats, and how specific diets such as **high-fat, low-carb**, and **Mediterranean** can promote hormonal harmony.

The Role of Macronutrients in Hormonal Health

Macronutrients—proteins, carbohydrates, and fats—are the building blocks for many essential processes in the body, including hormone production and balance. Each macronutrient plays a unique role in supporting hormonal health, and understanding how to balance them in your diet is crucial for maintaining stable hormone levels.

1. Proteins: Building Blocks of Hormones

Proteins are more than just muscle builders. They are fundamental to the production of hormones that regulate metabolism, growth, and stress responses. Proteins are broken down into **amino acids**, which are the raw materials for producing hormones like **insulin**, **growth hormone**, and **thyroid hormones**.

- **Insulin and Protein**: Insulin, produced by the pancreas, helps regulate blood sugar by allowing cells to absorb glucose. Protein, especially when paired with other macronutrients, plays a key role in stabilizing blood sugar and promoting **insulin sensitivity**, making it easier for cells to use insulin effectively. High-quality protein from sources like **chicken**, **eggs**, **fish**, and **legumes** helps prevent insulin resistance, a condition that occurs when the body becomes less responsive to insulin, which can lead to **type 2 diabetes** and weight gain.

- **Thyroid Hormones and Protein**: The thyroid, which produces **T3** and **T4** hormones responsible for regulating metabolism, relies on certain amino acids, especially **tyrosine**, to function properly. Without adequate protein intake, thyroid hormone production may decline, leading to **hypothyroidism** (underactive thyroid), which causes fatigue, weight gain, and cognitive issues. A **2019 study** published in *The American Journal of Clinical Nutrition* found that participants who consumed a higher-protein diet showed improvements in insulin sensitivity and thyroid function compared to those on a low-protein diet. This highlights how critical protein is in maintaining hormonal balance, particularly when it comes to insulin and thyroid health.

2. Carbohydrates: Fuel for Energy and Hormonal Stability

Carbohydrates are the body's primary energy source, but the type of carbohydrates you consume plays a major role in hormone regulation. The quality of carbohydrates in your diet directly affects how well your body manages blood sugar and hormone levels, especially **insulin** and **estrogen**.

- **Simple vs. Complex Carbohydrates**: Simple carbohydrates, such as **white bread**, **sugary snacks**, and **pastries**, are quickly digested and cause rapid spikes in blood sugar. This leads to a surge of insulin to manage the glucose in the bloodstream. Over time, these insulin spikes can cause **insulin resistance**, which not only affects metabolism but also influences **estrogen** production. High insulin levels can stimulate increased estrogen production, contributing to conditions like **premenstrual syndrome (PMS), polycystic ovary syndrome (PCOS)**, and **estrogen dominance**.

In contrast, **complex carbohydrates**—like whole grains, vegetables, and legumes—are digested slowly, providing a more stable release of energy and promoting healthy blood sugar levels. These carbs are also rich in **fiber**, which plays a role in estrogen metabolism. Fiber helps the body eliminate excess estrogen, reducing the risk of estrogen dominance and hormone-related conditions. A **2020 study** in *The Journal of Endocrinology* found that women who consumed diets high in refined carbohydrates had significantly higher levels of circulating estrogen and an increased risk of estrogen-dependent conditions like **endometriosis** and **breast cancer**. On the other hand, women who consumed complex carbs with plenty of fiber saw improved estrogen metabolism and reduced hormonal symptoms.

3. Fats: Crucial for Hormone Production

Fats are vital for the production of hormones, especially **steroid hormones** such as estrogen, progesterone, testosterone, and cortisol. These hormones are synthesized from **cholesterol**, a type of fat, and without enough healthy fats in your diet, hormone production can be impaired.

- **Healthy Fats for Hormone Balance**: Fats like **omega-3 fatty acids**, found in **fatty fish** (like salmon, mackerel, and sardines), **flaxseeds**, and **chia seeds**, play an important role in reducing inflammation and supporting the production of **prostaglandins**, hormone-like substances that regulate processes such as **inflammation** and **menstrual cramps**. Omega-3s are also linked to improved hormone regulation, reduced symptoms of **PMS**, and enhanced fertility.

- **Saturated Fats and Hormone Synthesis**: Despite their bad reputation, **saturated fats** from high-quality sources, such as **grass-fed butter** and **coconut oil**, are necessary for hormone production. Cholesterol derived from these fats serves as the precursor for many hormones. However, it's essential to differentiate between healthy sources of fats and **trans fats** or processed fats, which can harm hormone production and increase inflammation. A **2018 study** in *The Journal of Lipid Research* concluded that women who consumed healthy fats, including omega-3s and moderate saturated fats, had more stable hormone levels, less inflammation, and a lower risk of insulin resistance compared to those who consumed diets high in trans fats.

How Sugar, Refined Carbohydrates, and Unhealthy Fats Disrupt Hormonal Balance

While we've discussed how macronutrients can support hormonal health, it's important to understand how certain foods—like sugar, refined carbohydrates, and unhealthy fats—can disrupt the body's hormonal harmony. These disruptions can lead to conditions such as **insulin resistance**, **estrogen dominance**, and **chronic inflammation**, all of which have far-reaching effects on overall health.

1. Sugar and Insulin Resistance

Excess sugar is one of the most common disruptors of insulin balance. Eating too much sugar causes blood sugar levels to spike, leading to an overproduction of insulin to help bring glucose levels down. Over time, this can cause the body's cells to become **insulin-resistant**, forcing the pancreas to produce even more insulin.

- **Insulin Spikes and Resistance**: Frequent consumption of sugary foods and drinks can overwhelm the body's ability to manage blood sugar, leading to **insulin resistance**. When insulin resistance sets in, the body struggles to metabolize sugar efficiently, which can contribute to **weight gain**, **fatigue**, and even **type 2 diabetes**. Insulin resistance also affects other hormones, particularly **cortisol** and **estrogen**.

For example, studies have shown that high insulin levels stimulate **cortisol production**, which in turn leads to increased inflammation and stress in the body. Elevated insulin also encourages the production of estrogen, contributing to conditions like **PCOS** and **menstrual irregularities**. A **2021 study** published in *Diabetes Care* revealed that individuals who consumed high-sugar diets had a **30% higher risk of developing insulin resistance** and a **40% higher likelihood of developing type 2 diabetes**. The study emphasized the importance of reducing sugar intake to improve insulin regulation and prevent hormone-related conditions.

2. Refined Carbohydrates and Estrogen Dominance

Refined carbohydrates, such as **white bread**, **pasta**, and **pastries**, are stripped of their fiber and nutrients, leading to rapid digestion and insulin spikes. These insulin surges not only affect blood sugar but also influence estrogen production.

- **Estrogen Dominance and Refined Carbs**: High insulin levels stimulate an increase in estrogen production, which can lead to **estrogen dominance**. This hormonal imbalance occurs when estrogen levels are too high relative to progesterone and can cause symptoms like **bloating**, **mood swings**, **weight gain**, and **breast tenderness**.

Women who consume a diet high in refined carbohydrates are more likely to experience estrogen dominance, which increases the risk of conditions such as **uterine fibroids**, **endometriosis**, and **breast cancer**. On the flip side, consuming whole grains and fiber-rich foods supports estrogen metabolism and helps the body eliminate excess estrogen.

3. Unhealthy Fats and Hormonal Imbalances

While healthy fats are essential for hormone production, **trans fats** and **processed oils** can disrupt hormone synthesis and contribute to inflammation. These unhealthy fats are often found in fried foods, processed snacks, and fast food, and they interfere with the body's ability to produce and regulate hormones like **cortisol**, **insulin**, and **progesterone**.

- **Trans Fats and Inflammation**: Trans fats can disrupt the production of key hormones by blocking the body's ability to use **cholesterol** effectively. This leads to increased inflammation and hormonal imbalances, raising the risk of metabolic conditions like **type 2 diabetes**, **PCOS**, and **fertility issues**. A **2016 study** published in *The American Journal of Clinical Nutrition* found that people who consumed a diet high in trans fats were **50% more likely** to develop hormone-related imbalances, such as elevated cortisol levels and reduced progesterone production.

How Certain Diets Support Hormonal Balance

While individual foods impact hormone health, the overall dietary pattern is equally important. Specific diets, such as **high-fat, low-carb diets** and the **Mediterranean diet**, have been shown to promote hormonal balance and reduce the risk of hormone-related conditions.

1. High-Fat, Low-Carb Diets

High-fat, low-carb diets, such as the **ketogenic diet**, have become popular for their ability to promote weight loss and improve metabolic health. These diets emphasize healthy fats, moderate protein, and very few carbohydrates, helping to stabilize blood sugar and support insulin sensitivity.

- **Insulin Sensitivity and Ketosis**: By reducing carbohydrates, the body enters a state called **ketosis**, where it burns fat for energy instead of glucose. This process improves insulin sensitivity and reduces insulin levels, making it beneficial for people struggling with insulin resistance or hormone-related conditions like **PCOS**. A **2020 study** published in *Diabetes, Obesity, and Metabolism* found that participants who followed a ketogenic diet for 12 weeks experienced significant improvements in insulin sensitivity, reduced inflammation, and better hormone balance.

2. The Mediterranean Diet

The **Mediterranean diet** is often recommended for its anti-inflammatory benefits and its ability to promote long-term health. Rich in **healthy fats, fiber, whole grains, fruits, vegetables,** and **lean proteins**, this diet supports hormone balance in multiple ways.

- **Estrogen Metabolism and Anti-Inflammatory Effects**: The Mediterranean diet's focus on **omega-3 fatty acids, olive oil, nuts,** and **fish** helps reduce inflammation and balance estrogen levels. This diet also supports the body's ability to metabolize and eliminate excess estrogen, reducing the risk of estrogen dominance. A **2018 study** published in *The Lancet Diabetes & Endocrinology* found that women who followed the Mediterranean diet had lower estrogen levels, reduced PMS symptoms, and better fertility outcomes compared to women following a standard Western diet.

Conclusion: Using Food to Empower Your Hormonal Health

The food we eat plays an enormous role in supporting or disrupting our hormones. By understanding how macronutrients affect hormone production and learning which dietary patterns help maintain hormonal balance, you can take control of your health and prevent hormone-related conditions.

Balancing your intake of **proteins**, **carbohydrates**, and **fats**, while avoiding excess **sugar**, **refined carbs**, and **unhealthy fats**, is a powerful way to support your hormones naturally. Whether you choose to adopt a **high-fat, low-carb diet** or follow the **Mediterranean diet**, you are making choices that can positively impact your hormonal health, energy levels, and overall well-being.

Chapter 8

THE FOOD INDUSTRY'S ROLE IN HORMONAL IMBALANCE

HORMONES ARE COMPLEX AND delicate chemical messengers responsible for regulating everything from metabolism to mood, reproductive health, and stress responses. In recent decades, the food industry has significantly altered the way we eat, leading to profound implications for our hormonal health. The introduction of highly processed foods, artificial additives, and widespread use of chemicals has created an environment where many individuals unknowingly face chronic hormonal imbalances.

In this chapter, we will explore how modern food production, processing, and packaging contribute to hormonal disruption—specifically focusing on insulin, estrogen, cortisol, and thyroid hormones. By understanding the mechanisms at play and adopting practical solutions, you can take back control of your hormonal health and enhance your overall well-being.

The Influence of Processed Foods and Artificial Additives on Hormone Health

Processed foods have become a dominant feature of modern diets. From breakfast cereals and frozen meals to snack bars and sugary beverages, the convenience of these foods often masks the hidden costs to our health. But why do these foods disrupt our hormones, and how does it happen?

When we talk about processed foods, we refer to foods that have been significantly altered through industrial processing methods like refining, the addition of artificial ingredients, or preservation to extend shelf life. These foods may contain refined sugars, unhealthy fats, and synthetic chemicals that disrupt the body's hormonal systems.

Insulin: The Blood Sugar Regulator

One of the most immediate effects of consuming processed foods is the disruption of insulin, the hormone that regulates blood sugar. Insulin allows glucose (sugar) from the bloodstream to enter the body's cells, where it can be used for energy. However, many processed foods, particularly those high in refined carbohydrates and sugars, cause a sharp spike in blood sugar, which in turn triggers an overproduction of insulin.

Insulin Resistance:

This process of insulin overproduction leads to a phenomenon known as insulin resistance. When your cells are exposed to high insulin levels frequently—often due to a diet heavy in sugary foods and simple carbohydrates—they begin to become "numb" to insulin's effects. In a sense, your body stops responding to insulin's signal to absorb glucose, which leads to persistently elevated blood sugar levels.

Research has shown that insulin resistance is a precursor to various chronic health issues, including metabolic syndrome, type 2 diabetes, and obesity. It's important to note that insulin resistance doesn't happen overnight; it is the result of prolonged exposure to processed foods and refined sugars. In fact, it's estimated that 1 in 3 adults in the United States already has some degree of insulin resistance, making this a widespread but often overlooked problem.

Imagine you're setting off an alarm repeatedly—eventually, your neighbors stop responding. That's what happens to your cells when bombarded with excess insulin. At first, they respond by taking in glucose, but over time, they become resistant, leaving you with elevated insulin and blood sugar levels, creating the perfect environment for metabolic chaos.

Estrogen: The Female Hormone

Estrogen is often referred to as the "female hormone" because it plays a vital role in regulating the reproductive system in women. However, men also need balanced estrogen levels for proper health, including mood regulation, bone density, and cardiovascular function. The problem arises when estrogen levels become too high or too low, which can be influenced by the consumption of processed foods and artificial additives.

Many additives in processed foods, such as preservatives, dyes, and emulsifiers, have been found to act as **endocrine disruptors**. These are chemicals that interfere with the normal functioning of hormones in the body, often by mimicking or blocking hormone signals. One group of chemicals, known as **xenoestrogens**, is particularly concerning because they mimic estrogen in the body and can lead to a condition called **estrogen dominance**.

Estrogen Dominance:

When estrogen levels are disproportionately high relative to other hormones, such as progesterone, it can lead to a wide range of symptoms, including weight gain (particularly around the hips and thighs), mood swings, irregular menstrual cycles, and an increased risk of breast and ovarian cancers.

Consider the preservatives and emulsifiers found in many processed foods. These chemicals can act as xenoestrogens, which are foreign compounds that mimic the effects of estrogen in the body. Over time, regular exposure to these chemicals can contribute to estrogen dominance, creating a hormonal imbalance that disrupts everything from fertility to metabolic health.

Cortisol: The Stress Hormone

Cortisol, often called the "stress hormone," is essential for managing your body's response to stress. It helps regulate metabolism, control blood sugar levels, and reduce inflammation. However, when cortisol levels remain elevated for extended periods—as often happens with chronic stress or poor diet—this hormone can do more harm than good.

Processed foods, particularly those high in sugars and unhealthy fats, have been shown to increase cortisol levels. Research indicates that high sugar intake triggers the release of cortisol, and when consumed regularly, it can keep cortisol levels chronically elevated.

Adrenal Fatigue:

When cortisol levels remain high for too long, your adrenal glands (the organs responsible for cortisol production) can become overworked, leading to a condition known as **adrenal fatigue**. Adrenal fatigue can result in symptoms such as low energy, irritability, difficulty sleeping, and weight gain—particularly around the abdomen, which is often linked to high cortisol levels.

Cortisol is meant to help you deal with immediate stressors—like running away from a predator—but in today's fast-paced world, where stress is constant, and processed foods are a dietary staple, cortisol levels often remain elevated. This chronic stress response disrupts your hormonal balance and contributes to weight gain, mood disorders, and metabolic issues.

Endocrine Disruptors in Food Packaging

While much attention is given to the foods we eat, the packaging that those foods come in is equally important to consider. Many food and beverage containers contain **endocrine-disrupting chemicals (EDCs)** that can leach into the food, particularly when exposed to heat or prolonged storage. Two of the most common endocrine disruptors in food packaging are **Bisphenol A (BPA)** and **phthalates**.

BPA and Estrogen Disruption

BPA is a synthetic chemical used in the production of plastics and is commonly found in the linings of canned foods and in plastic food containers. One of the most concerning aspects of BPA is its ability to mimic estrogen in the body. BPA binds to estrogen receptors and interferes with the normal functioning of estrogen, leading to hormonal imbalances.

Health Implications of BPA Exposure:

Studies have linked BPA exposure to various health issues, particularly those related to reproductive health. Women exposed to higher levels of BPA have been found to be at greater risk for conditions such as polycystic ovary syndrome (PCOS), infertility, and breast cancer. In men, BPA exposure has been linked to reduced sperm count and altered hormone levels.

Consider how often you consume food from plastic containers or canned goods. Even small, repeated exposures to BPA can accumulate over time, leading to a significant hormonal imbalance. The problem is widespread, with studies detecting BPA in the urine of more than 90% of the population, a stark reminder of how pervasive this chemical is in our daily lives.

Phthalates and Thyroid Hormone Disruption

Phthalates are another class of chemicals used to make plastics more flexible. They are commonly found in food packaging, plastic wraps, and even some personal care products. Like BPA, phthalates can leach into food, especially when heated. Phthalates have been shown to disrupt **thyroid hormones**, which play a critical role in regulating metabolism, energy levels, and overall health.

Thyroid Dysfunction:

Thyroid hormones—specifically **T3** and **T4**—are essential for maintaining metabolic health, and any disruption to this system can lead to conditions such as hypothyroidism (low thyroid function) or hyperthyroidism (overactive thyroid). Studies have shown that exposure to high levels of phthalates is associated with lower levels of thyroid hormones, leading to symptoms such as fatigue, weight gain, depression, and difficulty concentrating.

Imagine your thyroid as the engine of your body. When phthalates interfere with thyroid function, it's like putting the wrong fuel in your engine—everything slows down, and your metabolism becomes sluggish, leading to weight gain and low energy levels.

The Effects of Pesticides and Chemicals on Hormonal Balance

In addition to the chemicals found in food packaging, the widespread use of **pesticides** and **herbicides** in agriculture poses another significant threat to hormonal health. These chemicals are often found on conventionally grown fruits, vegetables, and grains, and can remain on the produce even after washing.

Pesticides and Estrogenic Activity

Many pesticides contain chemicals that act as **xenoestrogens**—substances that mimic estrogen in the body. Long-term exposure to these chemicals through food consumption has been linked to an increased risk of **hormonal imbalances**, particularly in women.

Atrazine:

Atrazine is one of the most widely used herbicides in the United States, and research has shown that it can interfere with estrogen production. Atrazine exposure has been linked to reproductive issues, such as infertility and menstrual irregularities, as well as an increased risk of breast cancer. What's even more concerning is that atrazine has been detected in drinking water supplies, further increasing the risk of exposure.

Glyphosate:

Glyphosate, the active ingredient in many common herbicides, is another chemical with profound effects on hormonal balance. Glyphosate doesn't just kill weeds; it also disrupts an enzyme called **aromatase**, which is crucial for the synthesis of estrogen. By interfering with this enzyme, glyphosate can reduce estrogen levels in the body, leading to a host of reproductive and metabolic issues.

Glyphosate has also been shown to impact other hormones, such as insulin and thyroid hormones, making it a significant player in the development of **insulin resistance** and **thyroid dysfunction**. Given its widespread use in agriculture, glyphosate exposure through food is a growing concern for many people.

How to Minimize Exposure to Hormone-Disrupting Chemicals in Food

While it's impossible to eliminate all sources of endocrine disruptors from your environment, there are steps you can take to reduce your exposure and protect your hormonal health.

Opt for Organic and Non-GMO Foods

One of the most effective ways to reduce your exposure to harmful pesticides and chemicals is by choosing organic and non-GMO foods. Organic farming practices prohibit the use of synthetic pesticides, herbicides, and fertilizers, making organic produce a safer option for those concerned about hormonal health.

Why Non-GMO Matters:

Genetically modified organisms (GMOs) are often engineered to withstand heavy pesticide use, which increases the likelihood of chemical residues on your food. By opting for organic, non-GMO foods, you can reduce your exposure to glyphosate and other hormone-disrupting chemicals.

Choose BPA-Free and Phthalate-Free Packaging

When it comes to food packaging, look for products that are labeled "BPA-free" or "phthalate-free." Many companies now offer canned goods and plastic containers that are free from these harmful chemicals. However, it's essential to be cautious, as some "BPA-free" products use other chemicals, such as **Bisphenol S (BPS)**, which may also have hormone-disrupting effects. Whenever possible, choose alternatives like glass or stainless steel for storing and heating food.

Wash and Peel Your Produce

While it's impossible to eliminate all pesticide residues from conventionally grown produce, washing your fruits and vegetables thoroughly can significantly reduce your exposure. Using a scrub brush for firmer produce and peeling items like apples, cucumbers, and potatoes can help minimize your intake of harmful chemicals.

Cook at Home More Often

Processed and packaged foods are a major source of endocrine disruptors in the modern diet. By cooking at home, you have greater control over the ingredients you use and the quality of the food you consume. Preparing meals from whole, unprocessed ingredients can help you avoid artificial additives, preservatives, and other hormone-disrupting chemicals commonly found in pre-packaged foods.

Use Water Filters

Since many pesticides and chemicals like atrazine and glyphosate can contaminate drinking water, consider investing in a high-quality water filter to reduce your exposure. Filters that use **activated carbon** or **reverse osmosis** are particularly effective at removing chemical contaminants from your water supply, ensuring that you and your family have access to cleaner, safer water.

Taking Action for Hormonal Balance

Balancing your hormones in today's world requires mindfulness about the food you eat, the packaging it comes in, and the farming practices behind it. While the modern food industry presents many challenges, you have the power to make informed choices that support your hormonal health.

By opting for organic foods, reducing your consumption of processed and packaged foods, and choosing safer alternatives for food storage and preparation, you can significantly reduce your exposure to hormone-disrupting chemicals. It's important to remember that small, consistent changes can lead to big improvements in your health over time.

Balancing your hormones isn't about perfection—it's about taking informed action and making better choices that empower you to lead a healthier, more vibrant life.

Chapter 9

THE SUGAR-HORMONE CONNECTION

SUGAR IS OFTEN SEEN as a harmless indulgence, present in everything from our morning coffee to the snacks we reach for throughout the day. But behind this sweet taste lies a complex relationship between sugar and our hormones, one that can lead to significant health consequences when sugar consumption becomes excessive. The modern diet, rich in processed and sugary foods, is contributing to a growing epidemic of insulin resistance, weight gain, and hormonal imbalances that affect millions worldwide.

In this chapter, we will explore the intricate connection between sugar and our hormones, how sugar impacts key hormones like insulin, cortisol, and estrogen, and the long-term health effects associated with high-sugar diets. We will also provide actionable strategies to reduce sugar intake and improve insulin sensitivity, empowering you to take control of your health.

How Excessive Sugar Intake Contributes to Insulin Resistance, Weight Gain, and Hormonal Imbalance

Sugar, particularly in its refined and processed forms, is more than just empty calories. It plays a central role in disrupting the delicate balance of hormones that regulate everything from blood sugar levels to appetite and stress responses.

The Role of Insulin: Regulating Blood Sugar

Insulin is a hormone produced by the pancreas that allows your cells to absorb glucose (sugar) from the bloodstream to use for energy. When you eat foods high in sugar or refined carbohydrates, your blood sugar spikes rapidly, causing your pancreas to release a surge of insulin. In the short term, this helps to bring blood sugar levels back to normal. However, when sugar intake is consistently high, it forces your body to produce more and more insulin, leading to a condition known as **insulin resistance**.

Insulin Resistance:

When your body is flooded with insulin too often, your cells become desensitized to its effects, much like a person who becomes less responsive to loud noises over time. In this state, the cells don't absorb glucose as efficiently, leaving excess sugar in the bloodstream. To compensate, your pancreas pumps out even more insulin, setting off a vicious cycle. Over time, this leads to elevated insulin levels, higher blood sugar, and ultimately, insulin resistance.

Insulin resistance is one of the earliest warning signs of metabolic disorders, including **type 2 diabetes**, **obesity**, and **polycystic ovary syndrome (PCOS)**. But its impact goes beyond just blood sugar regulation; it affects how your body stores fat and regulates other hormones.

Weight Gain and the Sugar-Insulin Cycle

Insulin is also known as the "fat-storage hormone" because of its role in directing the body to store excess glucose as fat, particularly in the liver and adipose (fat) tissue. This is why excessive sugar consumption is closely linked to **weight gain**, especially in the abdominal area. When insulin levels are chronically high due to frequent sugar intake, the body is in a constant state of fat storage, making it difficult to lose weight.

The Sugar-Craving Loop:

Another problem with excessive sugar consumption is the cycle of cravings it creates. When your blood sugar spikes after consuming sugary foods, it is followed by a sharp drop as insulin works to bring levels back down. This blood sugar "crash" often triggers feelings of hunger and fatigue, leading you to reach for more sugary snacks to regain energy. Over time, this cycle leads to overeating, weight gain, and a deepening of insulin resistance.

In a way, sugar hijacks the body's natural hunger signals, making it easy to overconsume calories and challenging to achieve a healthy weight.

The Addictive Nature of Sugar and Its Effects on Cortisol and Estrogen

Beyond its role in insulin regulation and fat storage, sugar also has profound effects on other key hormones, particularly **cortisol** and **estrogen**. One of the reasons why it's so difficult to quit sugar is because of its addictive properties, which are deeply intertwined with the body's stress response and reproductive health.

Cortisol: The Stress Hormone

Cortisol is your body's primary stress hormone, released by the adrenal glands in response to both physical and emotional stress. While cortisol is essential for managing acute stress, chronically elevated cortisol levels can lead to numerous health issues, including hormonal imbalances, weight gain, and even insulin resistance.

Sugar and the Stress Response:

When you consume sugar, it causes a rapid spike in blood sugar levels, triggering the release of insulin. At the same time, your body perceives the sudden rise and fall of blood sugar as a stressor, prompting the adrenal glands to release cortisol to help stabilize the system. This is why sugar cravings often increase during times of stress—your body seeks out sugar to boost energy levels quickly, but the result is an elevation in cortisol that can exacerbate stress over time.

Over time, the combination of high sugar intake and chronic stress can lead to **adrenal fatigue**, where the body becomes less capable of producing and regulating cortisol effectively. This state of hormonal imbalance not only affects stress management but also plays a significant role in **weight gain**, particularly in the abdominal area, where cortisol tends to promote fat storage.

Estrogen and Sugar: A Delicate Balance

Estrogen, often regarded as the primary female hormone, plays a vital role in reproductive health, mood regulation, and even bone health. However, like insulin, estrogen is sensitive to dietary factors, particularly sugar. Excessive sugar consumption can disrupt estrogen balance, leading to conditions like **estrogen dominance**, where estrogen levels are disproportionately high relative to other hormones such as progesterone.

The Estrogen-Sugar Connection:

Sugar impacts estrogen levels in several ways. First, insulin resistance, which is often caused by high sugar intake, can lead to higher levels of estrogen in the body. This is because insulin resistance interferes with the normal balance of sex hormones. Women with conditions like PCOS, which is closely linked to insulin resistance, often have elevated estrogen levels and may experience symptoms like irregular menstrual cycles, weight gain, and mood swings.

Second, sugar consumption can increase the production of **xenoestrogens**, foreign chemicals found in processed foods and certain environmental toxins that mimic estrogen in the body. These xenoestrogens can further disrupt the balance of natural hormones, leading to issues like **infertility**, **PMS**, and an increased risk of estrogen-sensitive cancers.

Studies Linking High-Sugar Diets to Increased Risk of PCOS and Metabolic Syndrome

The connection between sugar and hormone imbalance is not just theoretical; it is backed by substantial research linking high-sugar diets to an increased risk of several hormonal disorders, including **polycystic ovary syndrome (PCOS)** and **metabolic syndrome**.

Polycystic Ovary Syndrome (PCOS) and Insulin Resistance

PCOS is one of the most common hormonal disorders in women of reproductive age and is characterized by irregular menstrual cycles, excessive hair growth, and ovarian cysts. One of the key drivers of PCOS is insulin resistance, which leads to elevated insulin levels and disrupts the normal balance of reproductive hormones.

Research Highlights:

Studies have shown that women with PCOS are more likely to have higher levels of insulin resistance compared to women without the condition. This makes them particularly vulnerable to the effects of a high-sugar diet. One study published in the journal *Fertility and Sterility* found that women with PCOS who consumed a diet high in sugar and refined carbohydrates had significantly worse insulin sensitivity and higher levels of androgen (male hormone) production compared to those who followed a lower-sugar diet.

Reducing sugar intake and improving insulin sensitivity through dietary changes and physical activity can help regulate menstrual cycles, improve fertility, and reduce other symptoms of PCOS.

Metabolic Syndrome: A Cluster of Risk Factors

Metabolic syndrome is a collection of conditions that occur together, increasing the risk of heart disease, stroke, and type 2 diabetes. It includes high blood pressure, high blood sugar, excess body fat around the waist, and abnormal cholesterol levels. Insulin resistance is at the core of metabolic syndrome, and high sugar consumption is one of the primary contributors to its development.

Research Highlights:

A study published in the journal *Circulation* found that individuals who consumed a diet high in sugar-sweetened beverages were significantly more likely to develop metabolic syndrome over time. The study highlighted that even moderate sugar consumption was associated with increased risk, suggesting that reducing sugar intake is critical for preventing and managing metabolic syndrome.

High-sugar diets also contribute to **non-alcoholic fatty liver disease (NAFLD)**, another condition often seen in individuals with metabolic syndrome. NAFLD is characterized by the accumulation of excess fat in the liver and is strongly associated with insulin resistance and obesity. Limiting sugar, particularly **fructose**, is a key strategy in preventing and reversing fatty liver disease.

Strategies for Reducing Sugar and Improving Insulin Sensitivity

Reducing sugar intake and improving insulin sensitivity are essential steps for restoring hormonal balance and improving overall health. Fortunately, there are several effective strategies that you can incorporate into your lifestyle to reduce sugar dependence and enhance your body's ability to regulate insulin.

1. Embrace Low-Sugar Alternatives

One of the easiest ways to reduce sugar intake is by substituting high-sugar foods with low-sugar alternatives. This doesn't mean giving up all sweetness—there are plenty of naturally sweet foods that won't cause the same spikes in blood sugar as refined sugar.

Some Low-Sugar Alternatives Include:

- **Stevia:** A natural sweetener derived from the stevia plant that contains zero calories and doesn't affect blood sugar levels.

- **Monk fruit:** Another natural sweetener that is hundreds of times sweeter than sugar but has no impact on insulin.

- **Fruit-based sweetness:** Whole fruits like berries, apples, and oranges contain fiber, which slows down the absorption of natural sugars and prevents blood sugar spikes.

Incorporating these alternatives into your diet can satisfy your sweet tooth without the negative effects on your hormones.

2. Practice Intermittent Fasting

Intermittent fasting (IF) is an eating pattern that cycles between periods of eating and fasting. Research has shown that intermittent fasting can improve insulin sensitivity and reduce the risk of insulin resistance. By giving your body a break from constant sugar and calorie intake, you allow your insulin levels to decrease, which in turn helps the body use stored fat for energy and regulate hormones more effectively.

How to Start:

There are various approaches to intermittent fasting, but one of the most popular is the 16:8 method, where you fast for 16 hours and have an 8-hour window for eating. During the fasting period, the body enters a state where insulin levels drop, and fat-burning hormones increase, helping to restore insulin sensitivity and support weight loss.

3. Focus on Whole Foods

Whole foods—such as vegetables, lean proteins, whole grains, and healthy fats—are naturally low in sugar and provide your body with the nutrients it needs to function optimally. By prioritizing whole, unprocessed foods, you can reduce your intake of hidden sugars commonly found in processed and packaged foods.

Key Nutrients for Hormonal Health:

- **Fiber:** Found in vegetables, fruits, and whole grains, fiber slows the absorption of sugar, preventing blood sugar spikes and promoting insulin sensitivity.

- **Omega-3 fatty acids:** These healthy fats, found in fish, flaxseeds, and walnuts, help reduce inflammation and improve insulin function.

- **Magnesium:** This mineral plays a critical role in insulin sensitivity and is found in leafy greens, nuts, and seeds.

4. Exercise Regularly

Physical activity is one of the most effective ways to improve insulin sensitivity. When you exercise, your muscles use glucose for energy, which helps lower blood sugar levels and improves your body's response to insulin. Regular exercise also helps reduce stress, which can lower cortisol levels and promote better hormonal balance.

Types of Exercise:
- **Aerobic exercise** (such as walking, running, or swimming) improves cardiovascular health and helps burn excess sugar.

- **Resistance training** (such as weightlifting or bodyweight exercises) builds muscle mass, which increases insulin sensitivity and promotes fat burning.

By incorporating both types of exercise into your routine, you can enhance your body's ability to regulate hormones and improve overall health.

5. Manage Stress and Sleep

Chronic stress and poor sleep are major contributors to hormonal imbalances, particularly when it comes to cortisol and insulin. When you're stressed or sleep-deprived, your body produces more cortisol, which can lead to increased sugar cravings and insulin resistance.

Stress Management Techniques:
- **Mindfulness meditation:** Helps reduce stress by calming the mind and lowering cortisol levels.

- **Deep breathing exercises:** Can reduce the immediate effects of stress and help stabilize blood sugar levels.

- **Adequate sleep:** Aim for 7-9 hours of quality sleep per night to allow your body to recover and regulate hormones effectively.

Conclusion: Taking Control of Your Hormonal Health

The connection between sugar and hormones is undeniable, and understanding how sugar impacts key hormones like insulin, cortisol, and estrogen is essential for achieving hormonal balance. By reducing sugar intake, embracing whole foods, and incorporating strategies like intermittent fasting and regular exercise, you can take control of your health and improve your hormonal well-being.

Balancing hormones isn't about perfection; it's about making informed choices that support your body's natural systems. By following the strategies outlined in this chapter, you can break free from the cycle of sugar addiction and create a lifestyle that promotes long-term health and vitality.

Part IV

Lifestyle Changes for Hormonal Balance

Chapter 10

Exercise for Hormonal Health

Exercise is one of the most powerful tools we have to influence our hormones and overall health. It's not just about burning calories or building muscle—physical activity plays a vital role in balancing hormones like **cortisol, insulin, estrogen**, and **thyroid hormones**. Whether you're dealing with stress, weight gain, or hormonal imbalances such as **PCOS** or **thyroid dysfunction**, incorporating the right types of exercise into your routine can be a game-changer for your hormonal health.

In this chapter, we'll explore how different forms of exercise—like **strength training, HIIT (High-Intensity Interval Training)**, and **yoga**—affect hormone levels, how physical activity can reduce stress and improve insulin sensitivity, and how to tailor your workout routine to address specific hormonal imbalances. By the end, you'll have a deeper understanding of how to use exercise as a tool to balance your hormones and support your overall well-being.

How Different Types of Exercise Affect Hormones

Each type of exercise impacts hormones in unique ways. Some exercises are more effective at reducing stress and lowering **cortisol**, while others are better for improving **insulin sensitivity** or balancing **estrogen** levels. Understanding how these activities influence your hormones can help you choose the right workout routine for your needs.

1. Strength Training and Hormonal Health

Strength training (or resistance training) includes exercises like weight lifting, bodyweight exercises, and resistance band workouts. It's known for building muscle and increasing strength, but its impact on hormones is equally significant.

- **Cortisol and Strength Training**: Strength training can initially raise **cortisol**, the body's stress hormone, due to the physical effort involved. However, over time, regular resistance training actually helps lower baseline cortisol levels, making your body more resilient to stress. A **2018 study** published in *The Journal of Strength and Conditioning Research* showed that individuals who engaged in regular strength training had lower levels of cortisol throughout the day compared to sedentary individuals.

- **Insulin Sensitivity**: One of the key benefits of strength training is its ability to improve **insulin sensitivity**. When you build muscle, your body becomes more efficient at using glucose for energy, which means less insulin is needed to maintain stable blood sugar levels. This is particularly beneficial for people with **insulin resistance** or **type 2 diabetes**. A **2019 study** published in *Diabetes Care* found that participants who engaged in resistance training twice a week improved their insulin sensitivity by 30% over a period of 12 weeks.

- **Estrogen and Progesterone**: Strength training can also help balance **estrogen** and **progesterone**, particularly for women going through **perimenopause** or **menopause**. As estrogen levels decline, muscle mass tends to decrease, which can slow metabolism and lead to weight gain. Strength training helps combat this by preserving muscle mass and supporting a healthy balance of these hormones. For women with **estrogen dominance** (common in **PCOS**), strength training can help by reducing fat tissue, which is where excess estrogen is often stored.

2. High-Intensity Interval Training (HIIT) and Hormonal Response

HIIT involves short bursts of intense exercise followed by brief periods of rest. It's known for being highly efficient, delivering maximum benefits in a shorter amount of time than traditional workouts. The impact of HIIT on hormones is profound, especially in relation to **cortisol, insulin,** and **growth hormone**.

- **Cortisol and Stress Reduction**: HIIT workouts trigger a short-term spike in cortisol due to the high intensity of the exercise. However, like strength training, HIIT helps lower cortisol levels in the long run, particularly by improving the body's stress response. In a **2017 study** in *The American Journal of Physiology*, researchers found that participants who performed HIIT for 8 weeks had lower cortisol responses to stress and improved mental resilience compared to those who performed moderate-intensity cardio.

- **Insulin and Fat Loss**: HIIT is highly effective at improving **insulin sensitivity** and promoting fat loss, especially **visceral fat** (the harmful fat around organs). By increasing your heart rate and boosting metabolism, HIIT helps your body use glucose more efficiently, reducing the need for excess insulin. A **2020 study** in *Metabolism* found that people who did HIIT for 12 weeks saw a 40% improvement in insulin sensitivity and a significant reduction in visceral fat, making it an excellent option for people with **insulin resistance** or those looking to lose weight.

- **Growth Hormone and Muscle Repair**: One of the added benefits of HIIT is its ability to stimulate **growth hormone (GH)** production. GH is essential for muscle repair and fat metabolism, and its levels naturally decline as we age. HIIT workouts have been shown to boost GH production, helping to maintain muscle mass and support fat loss. This makes HIIT a particularly effective exercise for both hormonal balance and overall body composition.

3. Yoga and Hormonal Balance

While strength training and HIIT are great for building muscle and improving insulin sensitivity, **yoga** excels at balancing hormones related to stress, like **cortisol**, while also supporting thyroid function and **reproductive hormones** like **estrogen** and **progesterone**.

- **Cortisol and Relaxation**: Yoga is well-known for its calming effects on the mind and body. It helps reduce **cortisol** levels by activating the **parasympathetic nervous system**, also known as the body's "rest and digest" system. This reduces the stress response and promotes relaxation. A **2018 study** published in *The Journal of Behavioral Medicine* found that women who practiced yoga regularly had significantly lower cortisol levels and improved markers of stress resilience compared to those who did not practice yoga.

- **Thyroid Function**: Yoga, particularly poses that focus on stimulating the neck area, can help support **thyroid function**. The thyroid gland plays a critical role in metabolism, energy production, and hormonal regulation, and yoga postures like **shoulder stand**, **plow pose**, and **fish pose** have been shown to improve circulation to the thyroid and enhance its function. A **2019 study** in *Complementary Therapies in Medicine* found that individuals with mild hypothyroidism who practiced yoga for 12 weeks saw improved thyroid function and a reduction in hypothyroid symptoms such as fatigue and weight gain.

- **Estrogen and Progesterone Balance**: Yoga is also beneficial for balancing **estrogen** and **progesterone**, especially during the **menstrual cycle, pregnancy,** and **menopause**. Certain yoga practices, such as **restorative yoga** and **pranayama (breathwork)**, help regulate reproductive hormones by reducing stress and promoting relaxation. For women with conditions like **PMS, PCOS**, or those going through menopause, yoga can alleviate symptoms by encouraging hormonal balance.

The Benefits of Physical Activity in Lowering Cortisol and Improving Insulin Sensitivity

One of the most important ways that exercise benefits hormonal health is by reducing **cortisol** levels and improving **insulin sensitivity**—two key factors in preventing and managing hormonal imbalances.

1. Lowering Cortisol Through Exercise

Cortisol is the body's main stress hormone, and while it plays an important role in responding to stressful situations, too much cortisol can lead to weight gain (particularly around the abdomen), fatigue, mood swings, and hormonal imbalances. Chronic stress can keep cortisol levels elevated, which in turn can trigger **insulin resistance**, **thyroid dysfunction**, and disrupt the balance of reproductive hormones.

- **Exercise as a Cortisol Regulator**: Regular exercise, particularly moderate-intensity aerobic exercise and yoga, helps lower cortisol levels and improve the body's response to stress. While high-intensity exercises like strength training and HIIT can cause a temporary increase in cortisol, the long-term effects are beneficial. Over time, your body becomes more efficient at handling stress, leading to lower cortisol levels throughout the day.

A **2020 study** published in *Psychoneuroendocrinology* found that individuals who exercised for 30 minutes a day, 5 days a week, had significantly lower baseline cortisol levels compared to those who did not exercise. This shows how consistent physical activity can help regulate cortisol and improve hormonal balance.

2. Improving Insulin Sensitivity

Insulin resistance—when the body's cells stop responding properly to insulin—can lead to high blood sugar, weight gain, and an increased risk of conditions like **PCOS**, **type 2 diabetes**, and **metabolic syndrome**. One of the most effective ways to combat insulin resistance is through exercise.

- **How Exercise Improves Insulin Sensitivity**: Exercise helps muscles use glucose more efficiently, which reduces the amount of insulin needed to manage blood sugar levels. Both **aerobic exercise** (like walking, running, or cycling) and **strength training** are effective at improving insulin sensitivity. When combined, these exercises provide even greater benefits for blood sugar control and hormone regulation.

A **2018 study** in *Diabetes Care* found that participants who engaged in a combination of aerobic exercise and strength training experienced a **30-40% improvement in insulin sensitivity** over 12 weeks. This improvement not only helped reduce blood sugar levels but also contributed to better overall hormone balance.

Tailoring Exercise Routines for Specific Hormonal Imbalances

Not all hormonal imbalances are the same, and the type of exercise you choose should align with your specific needs. Whether you're dealing with **weight gain**, **fatigue**, or **stress**, tailoring your exercise routine to target these issues can enhance your hormonal health.

1. Weight Gain and Insulin Resistance

If you're dealing with **weight gain** or **insulin resistance**, exercises that promote fat loss and improve insulin sensitivity are crucial.

- **Best Exercises**: Incorporate a mix of **HIIT** and **strength training** to maximize fat loss and improve insulin sensitivity. HIIT helps burn visceral fat (the dangerous fat around your organs), while strength training builds muscle, which improves your metabolism and increases glucose uptake.

- **Frequency**: Aim for at least **3 days of strength training** and **2 days of HIIT** per week, combined with **light cardio** (like walking or swimming) on rest days to keep your body active without over-stressing it.

2. Fatigue and Thyroid Dysfunction

For individuals dealing with **fatigue** or **thyroid imbalances**, moderate exercise that doesn't overexert the body is best. Overdoing it with high-intensity workouts can exacerbate fatigue and stress the thyroid.

- **Best Exercises**: Focus on **low-impact cardio** (like walking, cycling, or swimming), combined with **yoga** to support relaxation and thyroid function. Strength training is beneficial, but keep it moderate—focus on lighter weights with higher repetitions to avoid overwhelming your system.

- **Frequency**: Start with **3-4 days of moderate exercise**, such as brisk walking or gentle strength training, and incorporate **yoga** at least twice a week to enhance relaxation and reduce stress.

3. Stress and Cortisol Imbalance

If stress is a primary concern and you're dealing with **high cortisol levels**, exercise can be a great way to reduce stress and promote relaxation.

- **Best Exercises**: Focus on **low-intensity** activities that help reduce cortisol, such as **yoga**, **Pilates**, and **walking**. Strength training and HIIT can be beneficial, but avoid doing too much, as high-intensity exercises can raise cortisol if overdone.

- **Frequency**: Aim for daily movement, whether it's a **30-minute walk**, a **yoga session**, or **light strength training**. Consistency is key in keeping cortisol levels balanced, but don't overdo it with high-intensity workouts every day.

Conclusion: Exercise as a Key to Hormonal Health

Exercise is a powerful tool for regulating hormones and improving overall well-being. Whether you're looking to reduce stress, lose weight, or address specific hormonal imbalances like **insulin resistance** or **thyroid dysfunction**, the right type of exercise can make all the difference.

By understanding how different forms of physical activity affect your hormones and tailoring your routine to meet your body's specific needs, you can take control of your health and achieve greater balance in both your body and mind. Remember, it's not about overexertion or perfection—it's about consistency, mindfulness, and finding what works best for your unique hormonal profile.

Chapter 11

SLEEP AND HORMONES

THE RESTORATIVE CONNECTION

SLEEP IS MORE THAN just a time to rest—it's a critical period when our body works behind the scenes to balance hormones, repair tissues, and reset our metabolism. When we don't get enough quality sleep, it doesn't just affect our mood and energy levels; it disrupts the delicate balance of hormones like **cortisol**, **insulin**, and **growth hormone**. Over time, these disruptions can lead to weight gain, stress, and a variety of health issues.

In this chapter, we'll look at how sleep affects our hormones, how poor sleep contributes to hormone imbalances and weight gain, and the real impact of sleep deprivation on our metabolism. You'll also find practical tips on improving your sleep to support better hormonal balance and overall health.

The Critical Role of Sleep in Regulating Hormones

During sleep, our body's hormonal systems go to work, ensuring everything from our stress response to our metabolism runs smoothly. Some of the most crucial hormones are directly influenced by how well (or how poorly) we sleep. Let's take a closer look at the major hormones involved.

Cortisol: The Stress Hormone

Cortisol is our body's primary stress hormone. It follows a daily rhythm, rising in the morning to help us wake up and dropping off in the evening so we can unwind and prepare for sleep. When our sleep patterns are consistent, cortisol stays on track, giving us the energy we need in the morning and letting us relax at night.

But here's the problem: when sleep is disrupted or cut short, cortisol gets out of sync. Instead of tapering off at night, cortisol levels can stay elevated, making it harder to fall asleep and stay asleep. This high cortisol can lead to a cycle of **poor sleep and high stress**, which over time can increase inflammation, cause weight gain (especially around the belly), and make you feel constantly on edge.

Imagine trying to wind down after a long day, but your body's still pumping out stress hormones like you're in the middle of a hectic workday. That's what happens when cortisol doesn't drop as it should. It's like having your foot on the gas pedal when you're supposed to be slowing down for the night.

Insulin: The Blood Sugar Regulator

Insulin is the hormone that helps regulate blood sugar by moving glucose from your bloodstream into your cells. When we get enough quality sleep, insulin works efficiently, keeping blood sugar levels stable. But when we don't sleep well, insulin sensitivity can drop, meaning the body has to produce more insulin to get the same job done.

This lack of sensitivity is where things start to unravel. When your body becomes less responsive to insulin, blood sugar levels rise, and your risk of developing **insulin resistance** increases. Over time, this can lead to weight gain and even **type 2 diabetes**. It's a classic case of "too much of a good thing"—in this case, too much insulin—leading to metabolic issues.

Think of insulin like a key that unlocks your cells to let sugar in. When you're sleep-deprived, that key starts to get a little rusty, and your cells don't open up as easily. This means more sugar stays in your blood, leading to all sorts of problems.

Growth Hormone: The Repair and Rejuvenation Hormone

Growth hormone is responsible for repairing tissues, building muscle, and even helping you burn fat. The majority of this hormone is released while we're in **deep sleep**, especially during the first half of the night. When you get enough deep sleep, your body can repair itself, regenerate muscle, and optimize metabolism.

However, if you're skimping on sleep, your body won't produce as much growth hormone, which can lead to **poor muscle recovery**, **weight gain**, and **sluggish metabolism**. Growth hormone helps your body use fat for energy, so when you don't get enough sleep, it's like telling your body to store fat rather than burn it.

Imagine trying to build a house without all the materials you need. That's what your body is doing when you don't get enough deep sleep—it's missing the essential tools (like growth hormone) it needs to repair and rebuild.

How Poor Sleep Contributes to Hormonal Imbalances and Weight Gain

It's no secret that a lack of sleep can make you feel cranky and tired, but it can also lead to hormonal imbalances that contribute to **weight gain** and other health issues. Poor sleep affects nearly every hormone in your body, but the most noticeable impacts are on **cortisol, insulin,** and **hunger hormones** like **ghrelin** and **leptin**.

1. Cortisol and Weight Gain

When you don't get enough sleep, your body produces more cortisol. And while cortisol is necessary in small doses to help us deal with stress, having too much of it—especially at night—leads to **increased appetite** and cravings for sugary, high-carb foods. Over time, these cravings can lead to **weight gain**, particularly around the midsection, which is directly linked to cortisol.

Have you ever noticed how after a poor night's sleep, you're more likely to reach for a donut or a sugary coffee drink? That's cortisol talking. It's signaling your body to get a quick energy fix, which often leads to unhealthy food choices.

2. Insulin Resistance and Belly Fat

As mentioned earlier, sleep deprivation makes your cells less sensitive to insulin. This means your body needs to pump out more insulin to keep your blood sugar in check. The problem? High insulin levels lead to **fat storage**, particularly in the belly area. Over time, this can result in **insulin resistance**, where your body struggles to regulate blood sugar properly, increasing the risk of diabetes and metabolic issues.

In a sense, poor sleep makes it harder for your body to "burn off" food efficiently. Instead, it's more likely to store fat—especially in areas that are associated with **metabolic syndrome** and other health concerns.

3. Hunger Hormones: Ghrelin and Leptin

Two key hormones, **ghrelin** and **leptin**, are responsible for regulating hunger and fullness. Ghrelin increases your appetite, while leptin signals to your brain that you're full and don't need to eat more. When you don't get enough sleep, ghrelin levels go up and leptin levels go down, meaning you're **hungrier than usual** and less likely to feel satisfied after eating.

This is why poor sleep often leads to overeating and weight gain—your body is literally telling you that you're hungry, even when you've had enough food. It's like your hunger hormones are playing tricks on you, pushing you to eat more than you need.

The Impact of Sleep Deprivation on Hormonal Health and Metabolism

Sleep deprivation doesn't just make you tired—it wreaks havoc on your hormones and metabolism. Even a few nights of poor sleep can lead to **increased hunger**, **decreased insulin sensitivity**, and **higher cortisol levels**. Let's break down how this affects your body:

- **Metabolic Slowdown**: When you're sleep-deprived, your metabolism slows down. Your body becomes less efficient at burning calories, and instead, it starts storing fat. You may also notice that you feel more sluggish and have less energy to exercise, which further contributes to weight gain.

- **Increased Cravings**: Lack of sleep affects the brain's reward system, making you crave high-calorie, sugary foods. You're more likely to reach for quick fixes—like cookies or chips—when you're running on little sleep because your body is searching for an energy boost.

- **Hormonal Imbalance**: Sleep deprivation throws off the balance of several hormones, leading to issues like **insulin resistance**, **cortisol spikes**, and increased **ghrelin** (the hunger hormone). Over time, these imbalances can result in weight gain, poor stress management, and even an increased risk of chronic diseases like diabetes and heart disease.

Sleep Hygiene Tips for Improving Hormone Balance

Getting enough quality sleep is one of the best ways to keep your hormones in check. Here are some practical sleep hygiene tips to help you optimize your sleep routine and improve your hormonal health:

1. Stick to a Regular Sleep Schedule

One of the simplest ways to improve your sleep is by going to bed and waking up at the same time every day—even on weekends. This helps regulate your **circadian rhythm**, which controls your body's sleep-wake cycle and ensures that hormones like cortisol and melatonin stay balanced.

2. Create a Relaxing Bedtime Routine

Establishing a calming pre-sleep routine can signal to your body that it's time to wind down. This could include activities like reading a book, taking a warm bath, or practicing deep breathing exercises. Avoid stimulating activities—like watching TV or scrolling on your phone—as these can keep your brain alert when it should be relaxing.

3. Reduce Exposure to Blue Light

Blue light from screens (phones, computers, TVs) can interfere with the production of **melatonin**, the hormone responsible for making you feel sleepy. To improve your sleep quality, try reducing your screen time an hour before bed or use blue light-blocking glasses if you need to be on your devices late at night.

4. Keep Your Bedroom Cool and Dark

A cool, dark bedroom creates the ideal environment for sleep. Consider using blackout curtains to block out light and setting the thermostat to a comfortable temperature. A cooler room helps your body lower its core temperature, which is necessary for falling and staying asleep.

5. Limit Caffeine and Alcohol

Both caffeine and alcohol can interfere with sleep. Caffeine stays in your system for several hours, so try to avoid it in the afternoon and evening. While alcohol may help you feel drowsy initially, it disrupts your sleep later in the night, preventing deep, restorative sleep.

Conclusion: Prioritizing Sleep for Hormonal Health

The connection between sleep and hormones is undeniable. Sleep is essential for regulating cortisol, insulin, growth hormone, and other key hormones that keep your body functioning at its best. By prioritizing quality sleep and adopting good sleep hygiene habits, you can support your hormonal balance, boost your metabolism, and improve your overall health.

Remember, small changes in your sleep routine can lead to big improvements in your hormonal health. Whether it's creating a calming bedtime routine, sticking to a regular sleep schedule, or limiting blue light exposure, every step you take towards better sleep is a step towards a healthier, more balanced life.

Chapter 12

STRESS REDUCTION AND MINDFULNESS FOR HORMONE BALANCE

STRESS IS AN INEVITABLE part of life. Whether it's due to work, relationships, or unforeseen challenges, we all face stress in varying degrees. But what many people don't realize is how deeply chronic stress can affect our hormonal health. When stress becomes a constant presence in our lives, it sets off a chain reaction in the body that impacts everything from our **cortisol** levels to our **insulin**, **estrogen**, and **thyroid hormones**.

In this chapter, we'll explore how chronic stress leads to hormonal imbalances, particularly focusing on the role of **cortisol**. We'll also dive into the proven benefits of **mindfulness-based stress reduction (MBSR)** and other stress management techniques like **meditation, yoga, deep breathing**, and **journaling** that can help restore balance and improve overall well-being.

How Chronic Stress Triggers Cortisol Imbalances and Disrupts Other Hormones

When we experience stress—whether it's a minor inconvenience or a major life event—our body reacts by releasing **cortisol**, the main stress hormone. Cortisol is essential in small amounts, helping us deal with stress by increasing alertness, providing a quick burst of energy, and improving focus. However, when stress becomes chronic, the constant release of cortisol can wreak havoc on our hormonal system.

The Role of Cortisol in the Stress Response

Cortisol is produced by the adrenal glands in response to signals from the brain. It's part of the **"fight or flight"** response, which prepares the body to either confront a stressor or escape from it. When faced with a stressful situation, cortisol levels rise to provide the energy needed to react quickly. Blood sugar increases, muscles become primed for action, and non-essential functions, like digestion and reproduction, are put on hold.

But while this response is helpful in short bursts, it's not designed to be sustained over long periods. In cases of chronic stress—whether it's due to work pressures, relationship issues, or even financial strain—cortisol levels can remain elevated for extended periods, leading to a range of health issues.

Cortisol Imbalances: The Domino Effect on Other Hormones

Chronic stress leads to **cortisol imbalances**, which, in turn, affect other hormones in the body. Let's break down the domino effect:

- **Cortisol and Insulin**: One of cortisol's primary functions is to raise blood sugar, providing a quick source of energy. But when cortisol levels are constantly elevated, it keeps blood sugar high, forcing the pancreas to release more **insulin** to manage it. Over time, this can lead to **insulin resistance**, where the body's cells become less responsive to insulin, increasing the risk of **type 2 diabetes** and **weight gain**.

- **Cortisol and Thyroid Function**: Chronic stress doesn't just affect insulin—it also disrupts the balance of **thyroid hormones**. High cortisol levels can interfere with the production of **T3** and **T4**, the thyroid hormones responsible for regulating metabolism. This can lead to **hypothyroidism**, where metabolism slows down, causing fatigue, weight gain, and brain fog.

- **Cortisol and Estrogen/Progesterone**: For women, cortisol imbalances can also impact **estrogen** and **progesterone** levels, particularly during the menstrual cycle, pregnancy, and menopause. When cortisol levels are high, the body diverts resources from producing reproductive hormones to focus on the stress response. This can lead to **irregular periods**, **PMS**, and even **fertility issues**.

In essence, when cortisol levels are out of balance, it creates a ripple effect that disrupts multiple hormone systems, leading to a range of physical and mental health issues. It's no surprise that many people dealing with chronic stress also struggle with weight gain, low energy, and mood swings—all of which can be traced back to hormone imbalances.

The Effectiveness of Mindfulness-Based Stress Reduction (MBSR) on Cortisol and Mental Health

Now that we understand how chronic stress disrupts hormones, it's crucial to explore ways to manage stress effectively. One of the most researched and impactful methods for reducing stress and balancing cortisol is **Mindfulness-Based Stress Reduction (MBSR)**.

What is Mindfulness-Based Stress Reduction (MBSR)?

MBSR is an evidence-based program developed in the late 1970s by Dr. Jon Kabat-Zinn at the University of Massachusetts Medical Center. It's designed to help individuals manage stress through **mindfulness practices**, which involve paying attention to the present moment without judgment. MBSR combines techniques like **meditation**, **body awareness**, and **yoga** to promote a state of relaxation and reduce the physiological effects of stress.

At its core, mindfulness teaches us to step away from the "auto-pilot" mode we often fall into during stressful situations. Instead of reacting impulsively to stress, mindfulness encourages us to observe our thoughts and emotions, allowing us to respond with greater clarity and calmness.

How MBSR Reduces Cortisol Levels

One of the key benefits of MBSR is its ability to lower cortisol levels. Studies have shown that individuals who practice mindfulness regularly experience significant reductions in cortisol, which helps restore balance to other hormones as well. This is particularly important for those dealing with chronic stress, as lower cortisol levels can improve insulin sensitivity, thyroid function, and overall hormonal health.

When you practice mindfulness, you're essentially teaching your body to deactivate the stress response. Over time, this lowers baseline cortisol levels, making it easier for your body to handle stress without overreacting. It's like turning down the volume on the stress dial, giving your hormones a chance to recalibrate.

In addition to reducing cortisol, MBSR has been shown to improve **mental health** by lowering symptoms of **anxiety**, **depression**, and **burnout**. The practice of being present and aware helps calm the mind, reducing the mental strain that often accompanies chronic stress. It's a way of retraining the brain to handle challenges without triggering a constant stress response.

Mindfulness and the Brain: The Science Behind It

What's fascinating about MBSR is how it actually changes the brain. Studies using brain imaging have found that mindfulness practice increases activity in the **prefrontal cortex** (the area of the brain responsible for decision-making and emotional regulation) while decreasing activity in the **amygdala** (the part of the brain associated with fear and the stress response). This means that practicing mindfulness can literally reshape the way your brain responds to stress, making it easier to stay calm in challenging situations.

Practical Stress Management Techniques

While MBSR is an incredibly effective tool for managing stress, there are several other **practical stress management techniques** you can incorporate into your daily routine to help balance cortisol and other hormones. These practices not only reduce stress but also create a greater sense of well-being and emotional stability.

1. Meditation

Meditation is one of the most powerful tools for reducing stress and balancing hormones. It helps calm the mind, slow down breathing, and reduce the production of cortisol. By setting aside even just 10-15 minutes a day for meditation, you can significantly lower your stress levels and improve your overall hormonal health.

- **How to Start**: You don't need any special equipment to start meditating. Simply find a quiet space, sit or lie down in a comfortable position, and close your eyes. Focus on your breath as it moves in and out of your body. If your mind starts to wander (and it will!), gently bring your attention back to your breath without judgment. Over time, this simple practice can help you stay calm, even in stressful situations.

- **Types of Meditation**: There are several types of meditation you can try, including **guided meditation**, **body scan meditation**, and **mantra meditation**. Each one has its own benefits, so experiment with different styles to find what works best for you.

2. Yoga

Yoga combines physical movement with mindfulness, making it an excellent way to reduce cortisol and balance other hormones like estrogen and thyroid hormones. Certain yoga poses, particularly those that involve deep stretching and twisting, help stimulate the **parasympathetic nervous system** (the body's "rest and digest" mode), which lowers cortisol levels and promotes relaxation.

- **Best Yoga Poses for Stress Reduction**: Poses like **child's pose, seated forward bend**, and **legs-up-the-wall pose** are particularly effective at calming the mind and body. Incorporating gentle yoga into your daily routine can help ease tension, improve flexibility, and reduce overall stress levels.

- **Breathwork in Yoga**: Yoga also emphasizes the importance of **breathwork** (pranayama). Deep breathing exercises like **alternate nostril breathing** or **ujjayi breath** can activate the parasympathetic nervous system and promote a sense of calm.

3. Deep Breathing

When we're stressed, we tend to take shallow, rapid breaths, which can increase cortisol levels and make us feel more anxious. **Deep**

breathing exercises can help reverse this response by activating the body's relaxation system and lowering cortisol. These exercises are easy to do and can be practiced anywhere, whether you're at your desk, in your car, or lying in bed.

- **How to Practice Deep Breathing**: One effective method is the **4-7-8 breathing technique**. Here's how it works:

    a. Inhale through your nose for a count of 4.

    b. Hold your breath for a count of 7.

    c. Exhale slowly through your mouth for a count of 8.

4. Journaling

Journaling is a powerful way to process emotions, release tension, and gain clarity. By putting your thoughts on paper, you can create distance from stressful situations and reflect on your feelings in a safe, non-judgmental way. Journaling is also a great tool for self-awareness, helping you identify patterns in your thoughts and behaviors that may be contributing to stress.

- **How to Start a Journaling Practice**: You don't need to be a writer to benefit from journaling. Start by setting aside 5-10 minutes each day to write down your thoughts, feelings, and any challenges you're facing. You can also try **gratitude journaling**, where you list things you're grateful for each day, which has been shown to improve mood and reduce stress.

- **Prompts to Get You Started**: If you're not sure what to write about, use prompts like "What am I feeling right now?" or "What's been on my mind lately?" Let your thoughts flow freely without worrying about structure or grammar—the goal is simply to release whatever is weighing on your mind.

Conclusion: Empowering Yourself Through Stress Management

Chronic stress can be overwhelming, but by incorporating mindfulness and stress reduction techniques into your life, you can regain control over your hormonal health and well-being. Practices like meditation, yoga, deep breathing, and journaling don't just lower cortisol—they also promote a greater sense of calm, resilience, and emotional balance.

Remember, stress management isn't about eliminating stress altogether (which is impossible), but rather about changing how we respond to it. By making small but consistent changes to your daily routine, you can significantly improve your ability to handle stress and support a healthier, more balanced hormonal system.

Chapter 13

TOXINS, HORMONES, AND DETOXIFICATION

IN OUR MODERN ENVIRONMENT, toxins are everywhere—hidden in the food we eat, the water we drink, the air we breathe, and even the personal care products we use. These toxins, known as **endocrine disruptors**, can interfere with our body's hormonal balance, leading to various health issues ranging from weight gain to fertility problems and thyroid dysfunction. While we can't completely eliminate our exposure to toxins, there are steps we can take to support our body's natural detoxification systems and reduce our contact with harmful substances.

In this chapter, we'll explore practical, sustainable strategies for minimizing toxin exposure and optimizing our body's ability to detoxify naturally. We'll also debunk myths about quick-fix detox diets and look at how you can create a toxin-free environment for better long-term hormonal health.

Understanding the Impact of Environmental Toxins on Hormonal Health

What are Endocrine Disruptors?

Endocrine disruptors are chemicals that interfere with the body's hormonal systems. Unlike other harmful substances, endocrine disruptors mimic or block natural hormones, throwing off the body's delicate balance. These toxins can be found in everything from **pesticides** and **plastics** to **household cleaners** and **cosmetics**.

Endocrine disruptors are dangerous because even in small amounts, they can have profound effects on the body. For instance, they may mimic **estrogen** or **testosterone**, leading to hormonal imbalances that disrupt fertility, metabolism, and mental health. Exposure to these toxins has been linked to **thyroid issues, insulin resistance, breast cancer**, and even developmental problems in children.

The Body's Response to Toxins

When toxins enter the body, our natural detoxification systems—primarily the **liver** and **gut**—spring into action. These systems work tirelessly to process and eliminate harmful chemicals. But when we're exposed to an overload of toxins, whether through diet, environment, or lifestyle choices, our detox systems can become overwhelmed. Over time, this can lead to:

- **Chronic fatigue**: Toxins can burden the liver and prevent it from functioning optimally, leading to low energy levels.

- **Weight gain and hormone imbalance**: When the body struggles to detoxify properly, fat cells may store excess toxins, leading to weight gain and hormone disruption.

- **Digestive issues**: A gut overwhelmed by toxins may become inflamed, causing bloating, constipation, or "leaky gut," which can further complicate hormone regulation.

Recognizing the signs of a toxic overload—such as frequent headaches, unexplained fatigue, or persistent skin issues—can help you take steps to improve your body's detoxification processes.

Supporting Your Body's Natural Detox Pathways

While many detox programs promise rapid results, the truth is that your body already has powerful systems in place for detoxification. The goal should be to **support these systems** so they can work optimally. Two key players in the detox process are your **liver** and **gut**, and focusing on their health will enhance your body's ability to eliminate toxins effectively.

Liver Health: The Silent Warrior of Detoxification

The **liver** is often referred to as the body's detox powerhouse. It processes everything we eat, drink, or are exposed to and breaks it down into manageable substances that can be eliminated through urine or feces. When the liver is functioning optimally, it plays a vital role in balancing hormones by breaking down **excess estrogen** and other hormone byproducts.

However, if the liver becomes overburdened by toxins, it may struggle to metabolize hormones efficiently, leading to imbalances.

This is why supporting liver health is critical to maintaining balanced hormones.

How the Liver Detoxifies

The liver detoxifies in two phases:

- **Phase 1**: Toxins are broken down into smaller compounds. During this phase, free radicals are produced, which can be damaging if not neutralized.

- **Phase 2**: These smaller compounds are then attached to other molecules, making them water-soluble so they can be eliminated through urine or bile.

To support these detox pathways, you need a variety of nutrients and antioxidants. For example, **glutathione** is a powerful antioxidant that plays a key role in neutralizing free radicals during detoxification.

Supporting Liver Health Naturally

- **Cruciferous vegetables**: Foods like broccoli, kale, and Brussels sprouts contain compounds that enhance liver detoxification enzymes.

- **Beets and garlic**: These foods help stimulate the liver's natural cleansing processes, ensuring toxins are processed efficiently.

- **Green tea**: Packed with antioxidants, green tea boosts the liver's ability to detoxify.

- **Hydration**: Water is essential for the elimination of toxins.

Drinking plenty of water helps flush out waste products through the kidneys and urine.

Gut Health: The Body's Second Brain

The **gut** plays a crucial role in detoxification, particularly in hormone regulation. The **gut microbiome**—the community of bacteria living in your digestive system—not only helps digest food but also aids in the elimination of toxins and excess hormones. A healthy gut ensures that toxins and hormone byproducts are properly excreted. However, an unhealthy gut can lead to the **reabsorption of toxins** and hormones, exacerbating hormone imbalances.

Gut Bacteria and Estrogen Metabolism

The **estrobolome** is a group of gut bacteria responsible for metabolizing estrogen. A healthy gut microbiome ensures that estrogen is properly broken down and eliminated from the body. However, if the gut becomes imbalanced (a condition known as **dysbiosis**), estrogen can be reabsorbed into the bloodstream, leading to **estrogen dominance**.

Supporting Gut Health Naturally

- **Fiber**: Fiber is essential for moving waste through the digestive system. Foods like oats, flaxseeds, and leafy greens support regular bowel movements, ensuring toxins and excess hormones are eliminated.

- **Probiotics**: Probiotic-rich foods like yogurt, kefir, and fermented vegetables introduce beneficial bacteria into the gut, supporting digestion and detoxification.

- **Prebiotics**: Foods like garlic, onions, and bananas act as food for good bacteria, helping them thrive and maintain a healthy gut environment.

Debunking the Myth of Quick-Fix Detox Diets

There's a lot of hype surrounding detox diets—whether it's juice cleanses, extreme fasting, or restrictive eating plans that promise to "flush out toxins" quickly. But the reality is that while these diets may offer short-term results, they often fail to address the long-term health of your liver, gut, and hormones.

Why Fad Detox Diets Don't Work

Fad detox diets are typically designed for rapid weight loss or to provide a temporary sense of "cleansing." However, these approaches can often do more harm than good by:

- **Depriving the body of essential nutrients**: Extreme diets may lack protein, healthy fats, or fiber, all of which are critical for liver and gut health.

- **Causing blood sugar spikes and crashes**: Juice cleanses and fasting may lead to fluctuations in blood sugar, which can cause **insulin resistance** and disrupt hormone levels.

- **Slowing metabolism**: Overly restrictive diets can slow your metabolism, making it harder to lose weight in the long term.

Instead of focusing on short-term detoxes, the key to balancing hormones and supporting detoxification is adopting **sustainable lifestyle changes** that provide long-lasting benefits.

Sustainable Detox Strategies for Hormonal Health

- **Nutrient-dense eating**: Focus on whole foods rich in vitamins and minerals, especially those that support liver function (like cruciferous vegetables and leafy greens).

- **Intermittent fasting**: Rather than extreme fasting, a balanced approach like intermittent fasting can support the body's natural detoxification processes without depriving it of essential nutrients.

- **Adequate hydration**: Water is one of the most effective tools for detoxifying the body. It helps the kidneys filter waste and ensures toxins are flushed out regularly.

Real Ways to Minimize Exposure to Endocrine Disruptors

While supporting your liver and gut health is essential, reducing your exposure to endocrine disruptors in the first place can make a big difference in your hormonal health. Here are some simple, actionable strategies to minimize contact with these harmful chemicals:

Choose Clean Beauty Products

Personal care products like lotions, shampoos, and makeup often contain harmful chemicals such as **phthalates**, **parabens**, and **triclosan**. These chemicals can mimic hormones and disrupt the body's endocrine system.

Simple Substitutes

- Opt for **paraben-free** and **phthalate-free** beauty products.

- Choose products that are **fragrance-free** or made with natural, plant-based ingredients.

- Look for certifications like **EWG Verified** or **USDA Organic** to ensure you're using clean beauty products.

Eat Organic and Non-GMO Foods

Organic foods are grown without the use of synthetic pesticides and herbicides, which are known endocrine disruptors. Choosing organic produce can reduce your exposure to these harmful chemicals.

Focus on the Dirty Dozen

If going fully organic is too expensive, prioritize buying organic versions of the **Dirty Dozen**, a list of fruits and vegetables most likely to be contaminated with pesticides (such as strawberries, spinach, and apples).

Reduce Plastic Use

Plastics, especially those containing **BPA** and **phthalates**, can leach harmful chemicals into your food and drinks. These chemicals mimic hormones like estrogen, leading to hormone imbalances.

Simple Swaps

- Use **glass or stainless steel** water bottles and food containers instead of plastic.

- Avoid microwaving food in plastic containers, as this can cause more chemicals to leach into your food.

- Look for **BPA-free** labels on products, but remember that BPA-free doesn't always mean phthalate-free, so read labels carefully.

Improve Indoor Air Quality

Indoor air can be a significant source of toxins due to household cleaners, synthetic fragrances, and dust that accumulates over time.

Air Quality Tips

- Use an **air purifier** with a HEPA filter to remove airborne toxins and allergens.

- Choose natural cleaning products made with ingredients like **vinegar, baking soda,** and **essential oils**.

- Consider adding indoor plants like **snake plants, peace**

lilies, or **spider plants** to help purify the air naturally.

Bringing It All Together: Detoxifying Your Home and Body Naturally

Supporting detoxification and minimizing exposure to endocrine disruptors doesn't have to be complicated. With a few simple lifestyle changes, you can create a healthier environment that supports hormone balance and long-term well-being.

Holistic Detox Routine

Here's a simple weekly routine you can follow to keep your detox pathways working efficiently and minimize toxin exposure:

- **Daily**: Drink plenty of water, incorporate fiber-rich foods, and opt for organic produce when possible.

- **Weekly**: Include liver-supporting foods like cruciferous vegetables, garlic, and beets in your meals. Practice mindfulness and deep breathing exercises to reduce stress.

- **Monthly**: Do a "clean beauty" audit of your personal care products, replacing harmful products with natural alternatives.

- **Seasonally**: Consider deep-cleaning your home with natural cleaners and swapping out plastic storage containers for glass or stainless steel.

Conclusion: Empowering Your Detoxification and Hormonal Health

Detoxification is a natural process that your body is designed to handle. By making simple, sustainable changes—like choosing clean beauty products, eating organic foods, and supporting your liver and gut health—you can reduce your toxic load and protect your hormones. It's not about drastic cleanses or extreme diets, but about making mindful choices that will have a long-lasting impact on your overall health and well-being. Empower yourself with these tools, and your body will thank you with better hormonal balance, more energy, and improved vitality.

PART V

Navigating Hormonal Transitions

Chapter 14

MENSTRUAL CYCLE AND HORMONAL FLUCTUATIONS

THE MENSTRUAL CYCLE ISN'T just about your period; it's a dynamic, ever-changing process that influences almost every part of your life. From energy levels and mood swings to changes in appetite and weight, hormones like **estrogen**, **progesterone**, and **testosterone** are constantly shifting throughout the month. Understanding these hormonal fluctuations can give you insights into how your body works, why you feel the way you do, and, more importantly, how to work *with* your body rather than against it.

In this chapter, we're going to break down the phases of the menstrual cycle, explain how your hormones fluctuate, and how those changes impact your mood, and energy, and even how you relate to others. More importantly, we'll cover practical strategies—what to eat, how to move, and self-care tips—that will help you balance those hormonal ups and downs. And, I'll introduce you to **cycle tracking**, an empowering tool that can help you stay in sync with your body's natural rhythm.

Understanding Hormonal Changes Across the Menstrual Cycle

Your menstrual cycle can be divided into four main phases, each with its own distinct hormonal pattern. These hormones don't just influence your reproductive system; they have far-reaching effects on how you feel physically and emotionally.

Let's take a closer look at each phase and what's happening in your body.

Phase 1: Menstrual Phase (Days 1-5)

Your period marks the beginning of your menstrual cycle. During these few days, both **estrogen** and **progesterone** levels are at their lowest, which often explains why you might feel more tired, moody, or even a little less motivated.

- **What's happening**: Your body is shedding the uterine lining that built up during the previous cycle. It's a time of "letting go," and it can feel like an energy drain.

- **What to expect**: Cramps, bloating, and mood changes are common. Some women experience a sense of relief or clarity as their body releases.

How to support your body:
- **Nourish with iron-rich foods**: You're losing blood, so it's a good time to focus on replenishing iron. Think **spinach**, **lentils**, **red meat**, or even a hearty vegetable soup. It's about restoring what's being lost, which is why light, comforting

meals often feel best.

- **Stay hydrated**: Water helps alleviate bloating and flush out toxins. Sip on herbal teas like **ginger** or **peppermint** to soothe cramps and calm your stomach.

- **Move gently**: You don't have to hit the gym hard. **Walking**, **yoga**, or **gentle stretching** can help ease cramps and boost your mood without overexerting yourself.

Phase 2: Follicular Phase (Days 6-14)

Once your period ends, your body starts gearing up again. **Estrogen** rises, and you'll probably feel more energetic, clear-headed, and ready to take on the world. This phase can feel like a breath of fresh air, especially after the lows of menstruation.

- **What's happening**: Estrogen is building up to prepare for ovulation, and **FSH** (follicle-stimulating hormone) is working to mature an egg in your ovaries.

- **What to expect**: Higher energy, more motivation, and often a better mood. You might feel like tackling big projects or being more social.

How to support your body:
- **Fuel up with complex carbs and lean protein**: This phase is all about building, so feed your body nutrient-rich foods like **quinoa, sweet potatoes, avocados,** and **chicken**. You'll

need that extra energy for what's ahead.

- **Take advantage of your energy**: Now's the time to do more intense workouts. If you've been putting off trying **HIIT** or a **new strength routine**, this is the phase where you'll likely have the stamina and motivation to do it.

- **Support mental clarity**: Estrogen also sharpens your brain, so take advantage by tackling work or creative projects you may have been avoiding.

Phase 3: Ovulatory Phase (Days 14-16)

Ovulation is the big event of the cycle—your body is releasing an egg. **Estrogen** is peaking, and you might notice that you're feeling your most confident, sexy, and social during these few days.

- **What's happening**: The spike in **LH** (luteinizing hormone) triggers the release of an egg from your ovaries. Estrogen is at its highest, and **testosterone** also gets a boost.

- **What to expect**: Increased libido, heightened energy, and a desire to connect with others. You might also notice clearer skin and an overall sense of well-being.

How to support your body:
- **Light, fresh meals**: Your metabolism may slow down a bit during ovulation, and you might not feel as hungry. Focus on **light, fresh meals** like salads with **lean protein** and lots

of **leafy greens** to support hormone detoxification.

- **Maximize your workouts**: Your strength and endurance peak around ovulation, so it's a great time for activities that challenge you—whether it's a **run**, **weightlifting**, or a fun **dance class**.

- **Enjoy the social boost**: If you've been avoiding a social event or networking opportunity, now's the time to go for it. You'll feel naturally more confident and outgoing.

Phase 4: Luteal Phase (Days 17-28)

After ovulation, **progesterone** rises to prepare the body for a potential pregnancy. If no pregnancy occurs, progesterone and estrogen start to drop, leading to the well-known symptoms of **PMS**.

- **What's happening**: Progesterone dominates this phase, working to balance the effects of estrogen and prepare the body for menstruation. If pregnancy doesn't occur, hormone levels drop, triggering your next period.

- **What to expect**: Mood swings, bloating, fatigue, and food cravings are common as hormone levels drop, especially in the days leading up to your period.

How to support your body:
- **Comfort with complex carbs**: You're likely to crave carbs in this phase, and that's okay! Focus on **complex carbs** like

oats, **brown rice**, and **sweet potatoes**, which can help stabilize blood sugar and curb cravings.

- **Magnesium for PMS relief**: Foods like **almonds, pumpkin seeds**, and **dark chocolate** are rich in magnesium, which helps reduce bloating and mood swings.

- **Slow down your workouts**: This phase can be draining, so switch to more restorative exercises like **yoga**, **Pilates**, or even just a leisurely walk.

Practical Strategies for Hormonal Fluctuations

By paying attention to your body's natural rhythms, you can adjust your lifestyle to feel more balanced and in tune with your hormones. The key is understanding where you are in your cycle and making simple tweaks to your daily routine to match.

1. Eat According to Your Cycle

Your body has different needs depending on which phase you're in. By listening to these cues, you can support your hormonal balance:

- **Menstrual Phase**: Load up on **iron-rich foods** like leafy greens and lean proteins to replenish lost nutrients. Incorporate **anti-inflammatory foods** like ginger and turmeric to ease cramps.

- **Follicular Phase**: Focus on **healthy fats** like avocados and nuts to support hormone production. Complex carbs like quinoa and sweet potatoes will help sustain your energy levels.

- **Ovulatory Phase**: Keep it light with meals full of **fresh vegetables** and **lean proteins**. Your digestion might slow down, so opt for foods that are easy to digest.

- **Luteal Phase**: Don't resist those cravings—embrace **complex carbs** to manage them healthily. Magnesium-rich foods will help ease bloating and mood swings.

2. Tailor Your Workouts

Your energy and strength levels change throughout your cycle, so matching your workouts to your hormones can help you avoid burnout and get the most out of your fitness routine:

- **Menstrual Phase**: Restorative activities like **yoga** and gentle **stretching** will help you feel good without overexerting yourself.

- **Follicular and Ovulatory Phases**: Take advantage of your rising energy with **strength training**, **HIIT**, or a long run. You'll be able to push yourself harder during these phases.

- **Luteal Phase**: As your energy dips, switch to **gentler workouts** like Pilates, walking, or swimming. It's also a good time for **rest** if your body feels tired.

Cycle Tracking: An Empowering Tool

Tracking your cycle isn't just for fertility—it's a tool for understanding your body better. By logging your symptoms, mood changes, and energy levels throughout the month, you can start to see patterns and adjust your habits accordingly.

- **Why Track?** Knowing when to expect PMS symptoms, energy dips, or periods of heightened focus helps you plan your workouts, meals, and even your work schedule more effectively.

- **How to Track**: There are plenty of apps like **Clue**, **Flo**, and **Natural Cycles** that make it easy to track your cycle. You can log everything from your period days to mood swings, cravings, and energy levels.

Cycle tracking isn't just about knowing when your period is coming; it's about understanding your body's natural rhythm and working with it, not against it.

Conclusion: Embrace the Rhythm of Your Cycle

Your menstrual cycle isn't something to fight against—it's a natural rhythm that, when understood, can actually work in your favor. By paying attention to the fluctuations in your hormones and adjusting your diet, exercise, and lifestyle accordingly, you can feel more in control of your body.

Rather than dreading certain phases of your cycle, see them as opportunities to check in with yourself and make the changes that will support your overall well-being. And remember, your body knows what it's doing—sometimes, it just needs a little support to help you feel your best.

Chapter 15

Hormone Health and Skin, Hair, and Nails

Hormones are the body's chemical messengers, and their influence extends far beyond reproductive health or metabolism—they have a profound effect on the appearance and vitality of your skin, hair, and nails. Hormonal shifts, whether due to aging, stress, or underlying conditions, can cause visible changes in skin elasticity, hair thinning, and even brittle nails. The key to addressing these issues is to understand how hormones interact with your body and how to take proactive steps to restore balance.

In this chapter, we will explore how hormonal imbalances affect the health of your skin, hair, and nails, and provide actionable strategies for promoting optimal health in these areas. We'll also look at the research connecting hormones to common conditions like acne, hair loss, and nail weakness, and offer insights on the nutrients and lifestyle habits that can help you maintain a healthy, youthful appearance.

The Role of Hormones in Skin, Hair, and Nail Health

Your skin, hair, and nails are highly responsive to the state of your hormonal health. Hormones such as **estrogen**, **progesterone**, **testosterone**, **cortisol**, and **thyroid hormones** play critical roles in maintaining the integrity and appearance of these tissues. Let's break down how each of these hormones influences your skin, hair, and nails, and what happens when they become imbalanced.

1. Estrogen: The Fountain of Youth for Skin

Estrogen is often called the "fountain of youth" hormone for its protective role in maintaining skin elasticity, hydration, and thickness. It stimulates collagen production, which is essential for keeping the skin firm and youthful. Estrogen also promotes moisture retention, giving the skin its plump, dewy appearance. This is why, during the reproductive years, many women enjoy naturally glowing skin.

However, as estrogen levels decline with age—particularly during **perimenopause** and **menopause**—the effects on the skin become evident. Reduced estrogen leads to a loss of collagen and moisture, resulting in **thinner**, **drier**, and **less elastic** skin. This contributes to the formation of fine lines and wrinkles, as well as sagging.

Estrogen and Hair Health

Estrogen also influences hair growth. During periods of high estrogen, such as pregnancy, many women notice thicker, more lustrous hair. This is because estrogen prolongs the growth phase (**anagen phase**) of the hair cycle. However, once estrogen levels drop (such as postpartum or during menopause), hair may enter the resting phase more quickly, leading to increased shedding and hair thinning.

2. Progesterone: Balancing the Skin and Hair

Progesterone, another key female hormone, balances the effects of estrogen in the body. When progesterone levels are in harmony with estrogen, the skin and hair benefit from both hydration and balanced sebum production.

However, **low progesterone levels** can cause skin issues like dryness or acne due to unbalanced estrogen dominance. Progesterone also supports healthy hair growth by working with estrogen to maintain the **hair follicles**.

3. Testosterone and Hair Thinning

Though typically associated with male traits, **testosterone** plays a role in both male and female bodies. In women, it is present in lower amounts and affects skin and hair health, particularly when levels become imbalanced. Elevated testosterone, particularly in conditions like **polycystic ovary syndrome (PCOS)**, can lead to **excess oil production**, resulting in acne breakouts. Testosterone can also contribute to **hair thinning** by converting to **dihydrotestosterone (DHT)**, which shrinks hair follicles and leads to **androgenic alopecia** (female pattern hair loss).

For men, testosterone plays a significant role in hair loss patterns. High levels of DHT are a major factor in male pattern baldness, and testosterone can also contribute to **seborrhea** (excess oil production), which can clog pores and lead to acne.

4. Cortisol: Stress and Its Impact on Skin and Hair

Cortisol is the body's primary **stress hormone**, and while it serves an important function in responding to acute stress, chronic elevation of cortisol can have detrimental effects on the skin, hair, and nails.

Cortisol and Skin

Chronic stress and the resulting elevation in cortisol levels accelerate the skin's aging process by breaking down collagen and elastin, the proteins that give skin its firmness and elasticity. This leads to the formation of fine lines, wrinkles, and a loss of skin elasticity over time. Elevated cortisol can also exacerbate conditions like **eczema**, **psoriasis**, and **acne** due to its inflammatory effects.

Cortisol and Hair Loss

One of the most common effects of elevated cortisol is **hair thinning** and **hair loss**. Cortisol disrupts the natural growth cycle of hair by pushing hair follicles into the **telogen (resting)** phase prematurely, leading to **telogen effluvium**, a form of temporary hair loss triggered by stress. This can result in noticeable shedding, which may persist if cortisol levels remain high.

5. Thyroid Hormones: The Metabolic Regulators

The **thyroid gland** produces hormones (**T3** and **T4**) that regulate your body's metabolism, including how your skin, hair, and nails grow and regenerate. When the thyroid is underactive (**hypothyroidism**) or overactive (**hyperthyroidism**), these hormones become imbalanced, leading to visible changes in skin, hair, and nail health.

Hypothyroidism and Its Effects

In hypothyroidism, the thyroid produces too little thyroid hormone, which slows down your body's metabolism. This can result in **dry, rough skin, brittle nails**, and **hair thinning**. Hair may become coarse, dry, and more prone to falling out, while the skin loses its ability to retain moisture, leading to a rough, flaky texture. Hypothyroidism can also cause thinning of the **outer third of the eyebrows**.

Hyperthyroidism and Its Effects

Conversely, in hyperthyroidism, where too much thyroid hormone is produced, the metabolism speeds up. This can lead to **sweaty, oily skin, brittle nails**, and **excessive hair shedding**. While hyperthyroidism may not cause baldness, it can accelerate the rate of hair loss, leading to thinning over time.

Nutrients and Lifestyle Habits to Promote Healthy Skin, Hair, and Nails

While hormonal imbalances can significantly impact your skin, hair, and nails, the good news is that there are several lifestyle adjustments and nutritional strategies you can implement to support their health and appearance. Hormone balance, combined with proper nutrition, can help prevent or reverse many of the common issues caused by hormonal fluctuations.

1. Nutrients for Healthy Skin, Hair, and Nails

a. Collagen and Protein

Since **collagen** is the primary protein responsible for skin elasticity and hair strength, consuming enough high-quality protein in your diet is essential. **Collagen supplements** can also help support skin hydration and reduce the appearance of fine lines. Foods rich in amino acids, like **chicken**, **fish**, **eggs**, and **bone broth**, provide the building blocks for collagen production.

b. Omega-3 Fatty Acids

Omega-3 fatty acids, found in fatty fish like **salmon**, **sardines**, and **flaxseeds**, help reduce inflammation and support skin hydration. Omega-3s also play a crucial role in promoting healthy hair follicles and reducing hair loss caused by inflammation or hormonal imbalances.

c. Biotin (Vitamin B7)

Biotin is often touted as a key vitamin for hair, skin, and nail health. It strengthens keratin, the protein that makes up your hair, skin, and nails. Foods like **eggs**, **nuts**, and **whole grains** are excellent sources of biotin, and supplementation can be beneficial for those experiencing hair thinning or brittle nails.

d. Zinc

Zinc plays a critical role in skin health by promoting wound healing and reducing inflammation. A deficiency in zinc can lead to **acne**, **hair loss**, and even **nail issues** like white spots or slow growth. Zinc-rich foods include **pumpkin seeds**, **oysters**, and **beef**.

e. Vitamin D

Vitamin D plays a role in hair follicle cycling, and deficiency has been linked to conditions like **alopecia** (hair loss). Ensuring adequate levels of vitamin D—whether through sunlight exposure, diet, or supplementation—can help prevent hair thinning and support skin health.

f. Vitamin E

Vitamin E is an antioxidant that helps protect the skin from oxidative stress and supports hair growth by improving scalp circulation. Foods like **almonds**, **spinach**, and **avocado** are rich in vitamin E and can support overall skin and hair health.

Research Highlight: The Link Between Hormones and Conditions like Acne or Hair Thinning

The connection between hormones and skin conditions like **acne** or hair thinning has been well documented in scientific research. Hormonal fluctuations, particularly those involving androgens like **testosterone** and **DHT**, can lead to increased sebum production, clogged pores, and acne flare-ups. Similarly, elevated androgen levels contribute to **androgenic alopecia**, where hair follicles shrink, leading to thinner, weaker hair.

Acne and Androgens

Acne is often driven by an overproduction of sebum, the skin's natural oil, which is regulated by **androgens**. When testosterone or DHT levels rise—often during puberty, menstruation, or conditions like PCOS—the sebaceous glands produce excess oil, clogging pores and leading to acne. This is why many women experience acne flare-ups before their period or during hormonal shifts.

Hair Thinning and Hormonal Imbalance

Hair thinning, whether due to **androgenic alopecia** or **telogen effluvium**, is closely linked to hormonal fluctuations. Elevated levels of DHT in the scalp lead to a shorter hair growth phase and longer resting phase, causing more hair to shed. Telogen effluvium, on the other hand, is triggered by stress-related cortisol spikes, leading to temporary hair loss.

Practical Tips to Support Hormonal Balance for Skin, Hair, and Nail Health

1. **Manage Stress**: Since cortisol is a major factor in skin aging and hair loss, finding ways to manage stress is crucial. Consider incorporating **yoga, meditation,** or **deep breathing exercises** into your daily routine to help keep cortisol in check.

2. **Balance Your Diet**: A nutrient-dense diet that includes healthy fats, proteins, and plenty of fruits and vegetables can provide your body with the building blocks it needs for skin, hair, and nail health. Avoid processed foods and added sugars, which can exacerbate hormonal imbalances.

3. **Stay Hydrated**: Drinking enough water supports your skin's elasticity and overall hydration, while also promoting healthy nail growth and preventing brittle nails.

4. **Sleep Well**: Sleep is crucial for hormone regulation. Prioritize 7-9 hours of restful sleep each night to support balanced cortisol and melatonin levels, which in turn influence skin regeneration and hair growth.

5. **Consider Supplements**: If your diet is lacking in essential nutrients, consider adding supplements like **collagen, biotin, zinc,** and **vitamin D** to fill in the gaps and support healthy skin, hair, and nails.

In conclusion, your skin, hair, and nails are a reflection of your internal health, particularly your hormonal balance. By understanding how hormones like estrogen, cortisol, and thyroid hormones affect these areas, and by implementing the right lifestyle and dietary changes, you can take proactive steps to maintain vibrant, youthful skin, strong nails, and thick, healthy hair.

Chapter 16

Perimenopause and Menopause

As we approach midlife, we all encounter the unavoidable reality of **perimenopause** and **menopause**. For some, these hormonal shifts may come like a soft whisper—subtle changes that gradually transform their daily lives. For others, it can feel like a sudden storm, with symptoms such as hot flashes, night sweats, mood swings, and even weight gain hitting hard and fast. Whether these changes are gradual or abrupt, one thing is certain: the transition is inevitable.

However, the narrative around menopause doesn't have to be one of dread or discomfort. Understanding what's happening in your body can help you make informed choices that will allow you to approach menopause with confidence. The more you know, the better prepared you'll be to support your health during this time.

Perimenopause: The First Step in the Journey

For most women, menopause isn't an overnight change. The first signs begin in **perimenopause**, a transitional period that can start anywhere between your early 40s and mid-50s. Some women experience perimenopause for as long as 10 years before reaching menopause.

During perimenopause, your body begins to produce **less estrogen and progesterone**—the two main hormones responsible for regulating your menstrual cycle, among many other things. The decline of these hormones, particularly **estrogen**, is what drives the most noticeable changes. However, it's important to understand that these hormonal shifts are not linear. Estrogen levels fluctuate up and down unpredictably before they gradually decline toward menopause. This is why some months may feel "normal" while others may be marked by symptoms that make you feel like you're on a rollercoaster.

Common Symptoms of Perimenopause

While every woman's experience is unique, here are some of the more common symptoms of perimenopause:

- **Irregular periods**: One of the earliest signs of perimenopause is a change in your menstrual cycle. Your periods might become shorter, longer, lighter, or heavier. You may skip periods altogether for several months, only to have them return unexpectedly.

- **Hot flashes and night sweats**: These sudden bursts of heat, often accompanied by sweating and a flushed face, can be mild or intense and may occur during the day or night, disrupting your sleep.

- **Mood swings**: Just as hormonal fluctuations during puberty or PMS can lead to emotional ups and downs, the changes in estrogen and progesterone during perimenopause can trigger irritability, sadness, anxiety, or even bouts of crying.

- **Fatigue**: As hormones fluctuate, it's common to feel more tired than usual, especially in the latter half of the day. This can also be exacerbated by night sweats disrupting sleep.

- **Weight gain**: Many women experience a shift in fat distribution during perimenopause, with weight accumulating around the abdomen. This is due, in part, to estrogen's influence on fat storage.

What's key here is recognizing that these symptoms are your body's way of signaling the hormonal shifts happening internally. While frustrating, they're not permanent and can often be managed with lifestyle changes, dietary adjustments, and stress management strategies.

The Transition to Menopause: What's Happening in Your Body

Menopause is officially defined as **12 consecutive months without a menstrual period**. Once you've hit that milestone, you've entered menopause. By this point, your ovaries have stopped producing significant amounts of estrogen and progesterone, which leads to the end of your reproductive capability.

But menopause is more than just the absence of periods. **Estrogen**, one of the body's most important hormones, affects much more than just reproduction. Its role in maintaining **bone density**, **heart health**, **brain function**, and **mood** becomes even more evident as levels decline.

Symptoms of Menopause

The symptoms of menopause can vary in intensity, but many women experience a continuation of what they first noticed in perimenopause. However, the drop in estrogen during menopause is much more significant, leading to more pronounced effects:

- **Hot flashes and night sweats**: These continue to be one of the most common symptoms. For some women, hot flashes may last for years after menopause.

- **Vaginal dryness**: Estrogen helps maintain the moisture and elasticity of vaginal tissues. Without it, many women experience vaginal dryness, irritation, and discomfort during sex.

- **Decreased libido**: The decline in estrogen, along with other hormones like **testosterone**, can lead to a reduction in sexual desire.

- **Bone loss**: Estrogen plays a crucial role in protecting bone density. When levels drop, the risk of developing **osteoporosis** increases.

- **Mood swings**: The drop in estrogen can affect the brain's serotonin levels, leading to increased anxiety, depression, or irritability.

While these changes may sound daunting, the more you understand what's happening in your body, the better equipped you'll be to take proactive steps to manage these symptoms.

Why Estrogen Matters Beyond Reproduction

We often associate estrogen with the menstrual cycle and fertility, but it's much more than just a "reproductive hormone." Estrogen has wide-reaching effects on various parts of the body, including your **bones**, **heart**, and **brain**. This is why the drop in estrogen during menopause can feel so dramatic.

Bone Health

Estrogen plays a key role in maintaining bone density. After menopause, the rate at which women lose bone mass accelerates, increasing the risk of **osteoporosis**. This is why postmenopausal women are at a higher risk for fractures, particularly in the spine, hips, and wrists. Without the protective effect of estrogen, bones can become fragile, making it essential to take steps to maintain bone health during this phase.

Heart Health

Estrogen also has a protective effect on the cardiovascular system. It helps keep blood vessels flexible and promotes healthy cholesterol levels. After menopause, the risk of developing **heart disease** increases as estrogen levels drop.

Estrogen's decline can lead to changes in **cholesterol levels**, including an increase in **LDL (bad cholesterol)** and a decrease in **HDL (good cholesterol)**, which can raise the risk of **atherosclerosis** (the buildup of plaque in the arteries) and other heart conditions. For this reason, heart health becomes a major focus for women after menopause, and proactive measures can significantly reduce the risk of cardiovascular issues.

Brain Function and Mood

The brain is also highly sensitive to hormonal changes, particularly to estrogen. Estrogen has a direct influence on the production of **serotonin**, a neurotransmitter responsible for regulating mood, sleep, and appetite. As estrogen levels drop, many women experience changes in their mental health, including **mood swings**, **anxiety**, **irritability**, and, in some cases, **depression**.

Additionally, many women report experiencing **"brain fog"** or difficulty with memory and concentration during menopause. This is often attributed to hormonal fluctuations but can also be linked to sleep disturbances caused by hot flashes and night sweats. Addressing sleep quality and reducing stress can help mitigate these cognitive symptoms.

Managing Menopause Symptoms: The Role of Hormone Replacement Therapy (HRT)

For decades, **Hormone Replacement Therapy (HRT)** has been one of the most effective treatments for managing menopause symptoms. HRT involves supplementing the body with **estrogen**, **progesterone**, or a combination of both to alleviate symptoms caused by the loss of these hormones. It's particularly effective for managing hot flashes, night sweats, and vaginal dryness, but it also has broader benefits, including protecting bone health and improving mood.

However, HRT is not without its controversies. It became a hot topic in the early 2000s when the **Women's Health Initiative (WHI)** study raised concerns about the potential risks of long-term HRT use, particularly regarding **breast cancer**, **heart disease**, and **blood clots**. The study led to a significant reduction in HRT prescriptions and left many women wondering whether the benefits of HRT outweighed the risks.

Since then, additional research has provided more clarity, suggesting that the risks associated with HRT depend on a variety of factors, including **when treatment is started**, **the type of hormones used**, and **how long the therapy lasts**.

The Benefits of HRT

For many women, the benefits of HRT far outweigh the risks, especially when it comes to relieving some of the most disruptive menopause symptoms. Here are some of the key benefits:

- **Reducing hot flashes and night sweats**: HRT is highly effective at reducing the frequency and severity of hot flashes and night sweats, which can significantly improve quality of life.

- **Improving sleep quality**: By alleviating night sweats and regulating hormone levels, HRT can help women get better, more restful sleep.

- **Vaginal health**: HRT can restore moisture and elasticity to vaginal tissues, reducing discomfort during intercourse and preventing vaginal atrophy.

- **Bone health**: Estrogen plays a crucial role in maintaining bone density, and HRT can help reduce the risk of **osteoporosis** and fractures.

- **Mood stabilization**: For some women, HRT can improve mood and reduce the emotional ups and downs caused by declining estrogen levels.

The Risks of HRT

Despite its benefits, HRT isn't right for everyone, and there are potential risks that need to be considered. These risks include:

- **Increased risk of breast cancer**: Combined HRT (estrogen and progesterone) has been linked to a slight increase in breast cancer risk, particularly with long-term use. However, this risk diminishes after discontinuing HRT.

- **Heart disease**: Early concerns about HRT and heart disease were primarily associated with starting HRT later in life. More recent studies suggest that starting HRT in **early menopause** (before age 60) may actually have protective cardiovascular effects, whereas starting it later may increase the risk.

- **Blood clots**: HRT, particularly when taken orally, can increase the risk of blood clots, including **deep vein thrombosis (DVT)** and **pulmonary embolism**.

Making an Informed Decision

The decision to use HRT should be based on your individual health profile and personal preferences. If your symptoms are severe and significantly affecting your quality of life, HRT may provide the relief you need. However, if you have a history of **breast cancer**, **heart disease**, or **blood clots**, you may want to explore alternative treatments. Always discuss your options with a healthcare provider who can help you weigh the potential benefits against the risks.

Natural Approaches to Easing Menopause Symptoms

For women who prefer to manage menopause symptoms without HRT, or for those who want to complement their hormone therapy with natural approaches, there are a variety of strategies that can help. From **dietary changes** and **herbal remedies** to **lifestyle adjustments**, these approaches focus on supporting your body's natural hormonal balance and alleviating common symptoms.

1. Herbal Remedies

Herbal remedies have been used for centuries to alleviate menopause symptoms. Some of these herbs contain **phytoestrogens**—plant compounds that mimic the effects of estrogen in the body—while others help balance hormones more generally.

- **Black Cohosh**: One of the most well-researched herbs for menopause, black cohosh has been shown to help reduce the frequency and intensity of hot flashes and night sweats. It is thought to work by influencing serotonin receptors, although its exact mechanism is still being studied.

- **Red Clover**: Rich in phytoestrogens, red clover may help alleviate hot flashes and improve heart health. While the research is mixed, some women report symptom relief with its use.

- **Evening Primrose Oil**: Known for its hormone-balancing properties, evening primrose oil is often used to reduce breast tenderness and improve mood swings associated with perimenopause. It's high in **gamma-linolenic acid (GLA)**, a fatty acid that can support hormone balance.

- **Maca Root**: This adaptogenic herb is traditionally used in South America to help the body cope with stress and fatigue. Some studies suggest it may improve mood and libido, making it a useful tool for women experiencing a decline in sexual desire during menopause.

2. Dietary Changes for Hormonal Balance

What you eat can have a significant impact on your experience of menopause. Certain nutrients can help stabilize hormones, reduce inflammation, and support overall health during this transition.

- **Phytoestrogens**: Foods like **soybeans, flaxseeds**, and **lentils** contain plant-based estrogens that can mimic the effects of estrogen in the body. Incorporating these into your diet may help ease symptoms of estrogen deficiency, such as hot flashes and vaginal dryness.

- **Calcium and Vitamin D**: Bone health becomes a major concern after menopause, so it's essential to get enough calcium and vitamin D to maintain bone density. **Dairy products**, **leafy greens**, and **fortified plant milks** are excellent sources, and regular sunlight exposure can help your body produce vitamin D naturally.

- **Omega-3 Fatty Acids**: Found in fatty fish like **salmon, mackerel**, and **sardines**, omega-3s help reduce inflammation and support brain health. If you don't eat fish, you can get omega-3s from **flaxseed oil, chia seeds**, or **walnuts**.

- **Hydration**: Dehydration can exacerbate hot flashes and bloating. Drinking plenty of water throughout the day and limiting alcohol and caffeine intake can help manage these symptoms.

3. Lifestyle Adjustments

Beyond diet and herbs, certain lifestyle adjustments can make a huge difference in how you experience menopause.

- **Exercise**: Regular physical activity is essential during menopause, not only for maintaining a healthy weight but also for supporting heart health, bone density, and mood. Strength training helps combat bone loss, while activities like **yoga** or **walking** can reduce stress and improve flexibility.

- **Sleep Hygiene**: Night sweats and insomnia are common during menopause, but practicing good sleep hygiene can help. Keep your bedroom cool, avoid screens before bed, and establish a regular bedtime routine to promote restful sleep.

- **Stress Management**: Chronic stress can make menopause symptoms worse, so finding ways to manage stress is crucial. Techniques like **mindfulness meditation**, **deep breathing exercises**, and **journaling** can help reduce cortisol levels and improve mood.

Bringing it All Together: Navigating Menopause with Confidence

Menopause is a natural phase of life, but it doesn't have to be one filled with discomfort or confusion. By understanding the hormonal changes happening in your body, you can take steps to manage symptoms, protect your long-term health, and embrace this new chapter with confidence.

Whether you choose HRT, natural remedies, or a combination of both, the key is to listen to your body and make informed decisions based on your personal needs. By focusing on a **balanced diet**, **regular exercise**, and **stress reduction**, you can ease the transition into menopause and feel empowered to take control of your health.

Menopause is not the end of your vitality—it's a new beginning, and with the right strategies in place, you can thrive during and beyond this transition.

Chapter 17

Postpartum Hormonal Health

Pregnancy is an extraordinary time for a woman's body, but the transition after childbirth is often an equally powerful experience—especially when it comes to hormonal changes. After the baby arrives, your body embarks on a journey of recovery, healing, and rebalancing. But while the excitement of welcoming a new life takes center stage, there's another, often hidden drama playing out in the background: the hormonal rollercoaster.

In the postpartum period, your hormones shift dramatically, affecting everything from your **mood** to your **weight** and **energy levels**. This is a delicate time, both physically and emotionally, and understanding how these changes happen—and how you can support your body's return to balance—can make a significant difference in your recovery and well-being.

The Postpartum Hormonal Rollercoaster

Let's start by breaking down the hormonal shifts that happen after childbirth. During pregnancy, your body produces high levels of **estrogen** and **progesterone**—both of which play essential roles in supporting your baby's development and maintaining a healthy pregnancy. After delivery, these hormones drop rapidly, triggering a cascade of changes in your body.

These aren't just gradual declines; they're steep and sudden. Your body is shifting from a state of sustaining new life to a focus on **recovery** and **nourishment** (especially if you're breastfeeding). The thyroid gland, another critical player in hormone regulation, also goes through significant changes in the postpartum period, potentially leading to complications like **postpartum thyroiditis**.

Here's what happens with some of the key hormones:

1. Estrogen and Progesterone

During pregnancy, **estrogen** and **progesterone** levels rise to support the growth and development of your baby and to prepare your body for labor. **Estrogen** helps regulate the growth of the placenta and maintains blood flow to the uterus, while **progesterone** helps prevent premature contractions and supports the thickening of the uterine lining.

But within 24 hours after delivery, levels of both hormones plummet to pre-pregnancy levels. This sudden drop is responsible for many of the emotional and physical changes that new mothers experience. This shift can lead to the familiar mood swings, crying spells, and irritability associated with the "baby blues," which affect many women in the first two weeks postpartum.

- **What this means for you**: With lower levels of estrogen and progesterone, you may feel a sense of loss or emotional sensitivity. Your body is adjusting to the new hormonal landscape, which can feel overwhelming.

2. Prolactin

Prolactin is the hormone responsible for **milk production**. After childbirth, prolactin levels rise to support breastfeeding. Prolactin helps to establish your milk supply and encourages bonding between mother and baby.

However, higher levels of prolactin can also suppress **estrogen** production, which may lead to symptoms such as **vaginal dryness** and **low libido**. These are normal, temporary effects, but they can feel disorienting, especially during the first few weeks postpartum.

- **What this means for you**: If you're breastfeeding, the shift in hormones can cause physical discomforts, such as vaginal dryness or even delayed return of your menstrual cycle.

3. Oxytocin

Oxytocin, often referred to as the **"love hormone,"** plays a critical role in bonding with your newborn. It's released in large amounts during labor to help stimulate uterine contractions and continues to be released during breastfeeding, promoting a sense of connection and well-being between mother and child.

But oxytocin isn't just a bonding hormone; it also supports the contraction of the uterus after birth, helping to reduce postpartum bleeding and aiding the uterus in returning to its pre-pregnancy size.

- **What this means for you**: Oxytocin helps you feel more connected to your baby and fosters a sense of emotional bonding. However, fluctuations in this hormone can also contribute to emotional ups and downs.

4. Thyroid Hormones

Pregnancy puts significant stress on the thyroid, and some women may develop **postpartum thyroiditis**, an inflammation of the thyroid gland that can cause either **hyperthyroidism** (an overactive thyroid) or **hypothyroidism** (an underactive thyroid). In some cases, women may first experience hyperthyroidism, followed by a period of hypothyroidism.

- **What this means for you**: An overactive thyroid can lead to **anxiety**, **weight loss**, **insomnia**, and **heart palpitations**, while an underactive thyroid can cause **fatigue**, **weight gain**, **depression**, and **dry skin**. If you experience any of these symptoms, it's important to talk to your healthcare provider and consider thyroid function testing.

Research Highlight: The Link Between Postpartum Depression and Hormonal Changes

One of the most profound ways these hormonal shifts manifest is through emotional and mental health changes, particularly **postpartum depression** (PPD). While it's common for women to experience the **"baby blues"** in the first few weeks after delivery—marked by mood swings, anxiety, and crying spells—postpartum depression is a more serious condition that can linger for months.

Researchers have long believed that the sudden drop in estrogen and progesterone after childbirth is a major contributor to PPD. Estrogen, in particular, has a strong influence on **serotonin**—the neurotransmitter responsible for regulating mood. When estrogen levels plummet, serotonin levels may fall as well, which can lead to feelings of **sadness**, **hopelessness**, and **disconnection**.

It's important to note that postpartum depression doesn't just affect the mother; it can have a ripple effect on the entire family. Recognizing the signs early and seeking help is crucial for recovery.

Signs of Postpartum Depression

Postpartum depression is more than just feeling tired or overwhelmed. Symptoms can vary but may include:

- **Persistent sadness or feeling empty**
- **Difficulty bonding with your baby**
- **Severe fatigue or lack of energy**
- **Changes in appetite (either eating too much or too little)**
- **Feelings of worthlessness or guilt**
- **Withdrawal from family and friends**
- **Thoughts of harming yourself or your baby**

If you're experiencing any of these symptoms, it's important to reach out for support, whether through a healthcare provider, a therapist, or a support group. Postpartum depression is treatable, and early intervention can make a huge difference in recovery.

Practical Strategies for Restoring Hormonal Balance Postpartum

Now that we understand the hormonal shifts happening after childbirth, let's focus on what you can do to support your body as it recovers. The postpartum period is one of **healing, rebalancing**, and adjusting to a new normal. Here are some practical strategies to help restore hormonal balance and support overall well-being during this time.

1. Build a Support System

One of the most important steps in postpartum recovery is surrounding yourself with a strong **support system**. Whether it's your partner, family members, or friends, having people around who can help with daily tasks, provide emotional support, and give you breaks is essential.

- **Why this matters**: Emotional and physical support can reduce feelings of isolation and overwhelm, which are common during the postpartum period. Simply knowing that you have someone to lean on can lower stress levels and aid in hormonal regulation.

- **What you can do**: Don't hesitate to ask for help. Whether it's someone bringing over meals, helping with household chores, or simply giving you a few moments of rest, every bit of support counts. Postpartum doulas, therapists, or support groups can also provide valuable assistance.

2. Focus on Nutrient-Dense Foods

Your body has just gone through an intense process, and nourishing yourself with the right foods is crucial for recovery. Focus on **whole, nutrient-dense foods** that provide the vitamins and minerals needed to support hormonal balance.

- **Key nutrients to focus on**:

    - **Healthy fats**: Include sources like **avocados**, **nuts**, **seeds**, and **olive oil** to support hormone production.

    - **Protein**: Aim for **lean proteins** like chicken, turkey, fish, and plant-based options like lentils and chickpeas to help repair tissues and maintain energy.

    - **Fiber**: High-fiber foods such as fruits, vegetables, and whole grains help regulate digestion and can prevent postpartum constipation.

    - **Iron**: After childbirth, iron stores may be depleted, especially if there was significant blood loss. Replenish with iron-rich foods like **spinach**, **lentils**, and **red meat**.

- **Why this matters**: The postpartum period is demanding, both emotionally and physically. Nutrient-dense foods help restore depleted nutrient stores, support energy levels, and assist in balancing hormones like estrogen and progesterone.

3. Prioritize Sleep (as much as possible)

We all know that sleep deprivation comes with the territory of being a new parent, but getting enough rest is one of the most important things you can do to support your hormonal health.

- **Why this matters**: Sleep regulates hormones, particularly **cortisol** and **insulin**. When you're sleep-deprived, your body produces more cortisol (the stress hormone), which can throw off your hormonal balance and lead to increased feelings of anxiety and irritability. Poor sleep also affects **insulin sensitivity**, contributing to weight gain and fatigue.

- **What you can do**: While it's unrealistic to expect long stretches of uninterrupted sleep with a newborn, try to nap when your baby naps. Delegate tasks to others when possible and take advantage of any moments to rest.

4. Gentle Exercise to Rebalance Hormones

While it's important to give your body time to heal after childbirth, introducing **gentle movement** as part of your postpartum routine can support hormone balance and improve your mood.

- **Why this matters**: Exercise helps reduce stress and boosts **endorphin** levels, which can improve mood and energy. Additionally, gentle movement like **walking, stretching**, or **yoga** can promote circulation and help regulate hormonal fluctuations.

- **What you can do**: Start slowly with activities like walking or gentle yoga. Over time, as your energy returns, you can gradually incorporate strength training or other forms of exercise, but always check with your healthcare provider before resuming more intense physical activities.

5. Stay Hydrated

Proper hydration is often overlooked but is essential for maintaining hormonal balance, especially if you're breastfeeding.

- **Why this matters**: Water supports all bodily functions, including hormone production, digestion, and energy metabolism. If you're breastfeeding, staying hydrated is crucial for maintaining your milk supply.

- **What you can do**: Aim to drink at least 8 glasses of water per day, and more if you're breastfeeding. Herbal teas and coconut water can also help keep you hydrated.

Bringing It All Together: Reclaiming Balance in the Postpartum Period

The postpartum period is a time of healing, adjustment, and profound change. Understanding the hormonal shifts happening in your body is the first step in navigating this transition with confidence. By building a strong support system, nourishing your body with nutrient-dense foods, prioritizing rest, and engaging in gentle exercise, you can help restore balance and promote recovery.

Remember, every woman's postpartum journey is unique. Give yourself grace, ask for help when you need it, and know that these early weeks and months are just one phase in your larger journey of motherhood.

The hormonal rollercoaster may be intense, but with the right strategies, you can navigate it with strength and resilience, setting the stage for long-term health and well-being.

Chapter 18

HORMONAL IMBALANCES AND FERTILITY

HORMONES ARE THE BODY'S chemical messengers, orchestrating many essential functions, including the complex process of fertility. For many women, hormonal imbalances can present a frustrating and often heartbreaking barrier to conception. Understanding how hormones like **estrogen**, **progesterone**, and **thyroid hormones** influence fertility is key to regaining control and supporting reproductive health.

Whether you're actively trying to conceive, planning for the future, or simply looking to optimize your hormonal health, it's essential to recognize the delicate balance required for fertility. But the good news is that with the right information and lifestyle strategies, you can take meaningful steps to support your reproductive health.

In this chapter, we will explore the effects of **hormonal imbalances** on fertility, with a focus on the primary hormones involved. We will also cover evidence-based strategies to help you restore balance and optimize your chances for conception. By the end of this section, you will have a clear understanding of how diet, lifestyle, and stress management play a significant role in fertility.

Fertility is a complex and finely tuned system in the body that requires the proper balance of several key hormones. These hormones regulate essential processes such as ovulation, the menstrual cycle, and the preparation of the uterus for pregnancy. Three of the most critical hormones for reproductive health are **estrogen**, **progesterone**, and **thyroid hormones**. Any imbalance in these hormones can significantly affect a woman's ability to conceive and maintain a healthy pregnancy. Let's dive deeper into how each of these hormones influences fertility and what happens when their balance is disrupted.

1. Estrogen: The Growth Hormone of Fertility

Estrogen is often referred to as the "primary female hormone" because of its central role in the development and regulation of the reproductive system. It's involved in many aspects of fertility, from regulating the menstrual cycle to preparing the body for potential pregnancy.

Estrogen's Role in the Menstrual Cycle

Estrogen levels fluctuate throughout the menstrual cycle, peaking in the **follicular phase** (the first half of the cycle), just before ovulation. During this phase, estrogen signals the **ovaries** to produce and mature eggs (known as **follicles**). This maturation process is crucial for ovulation—the release of a mature egg that can be fertilized by sperm. At the same time, estrogen helps thicken the **uterine lining (endometrium)**, preparing it for possible implantation of a fertilized egg. This thickening is vital because, without a sufficiently developed endometrium, implantation cannot occur, and pregnancy cannot be sustained.

In essence, estrogen plays the role of the builder—ensuring the egg is ready for fertilization and that the uterus is prepared to nourish a potential pregnancy.

Estrogen Dominance

Estrogen dominance occurs when estrogen levels are too high in relation to **progesterone**. This imbalance is often caused by factors such as **chronic stress, excess body fat**, or exposure to **xenoestrogens**—chemicals found in plastics, cosmetics, and even certain foods that mimic estrogen in the body.

When estrogen dominates, it can lead to a number of fertility issues, including:

- **Anovulation**: This is the absence of ovulation, meaning no egg is released during the cycle. Without ovulation, conception is impossible.

- **Irregular Periods**: High estrogen levels can disrupt the regularity of menstrual cycles, making it difficult to predict ovulation and plan conception efforts.

- **Polycystic Ovary Syndrome (PCOS)**: Estrogen dominance is often seen in women with PCOS, a condition characterized by hormonal imbalances that lead to irregular periods, cysts on the ovaries, and difficulty ovulating.

Estrogen dominance also promotes the excessive thickening of the uterine lining, which can lead to heavy, painful periods and issues like **endometriosis** (where uterine tissue grows outside the uterus). This can further complicate fertility by causing pelvic inflammation and scarring.

Estrogen Deficiency

On the other hand, **low estrogen levels** can also impair fertility. Estrogen deficiency is commonly seen in women who are **underweight**, **over-exercise**, or experience significant **stress**. These conditions can suppress estrogen production, leading to:

- **Ovulatory Dysfunction**: Without enough estrogen, the ovaries may not produce or release an egg during the menstrual cycle.

- **Thin Uterine Lining**: Insufficient estrogen can result in a uterine lining that's too thin for implantation, even if ovulation occurs. This can prevent a fertilized egg from successfully attaching to the uterine wall, leading to early pregnancy loss or infertility.

In short, both too much and too little estrogen can disrupt the balance required for a successful pregnancy. Women with estrogen imbalances often struggle with irregular cycles, anovulation, or miscarriages.

2. Progesterone: The Hormone of Pregnancy

While **estrogen** is essential for getting the body ready for ovulation, **progesterone** is critical for maintaining a pregnancy. Once ovulation occurs, **progesterone** takes over, preparing the body for the potential implantation of a fertilized egg.

Progesterone's Role in the Menstrual Cycle

After ovulation, the follicle that released the egg turns into a structure called the **corpus luteum**, which produces progesterone. During the second half of the cycle, known as the **luteal phase**, progesterone's main job is to maintain the thickened uterine lining that estrogen helped build. If fertilization occurs, the developing embryo will need this nutrient-rich lining to implant and begin developing.

Progesterone also plays a key role in preventing **uterine contractions** that could dislodge a newly implanted embryo, giving the pregnancy the best chance of success. If no fertilization occurs, progesterone levels drop, signaling the body to shed the uterine lining during menstruation.

Low Progesterone Levels

One of the most common fertility problems related to progesterone is **low progesterone levels**. Without enough progesterone, the luteal phase may be shortened, and the uterine lining may not be adequately prepared to support pregnancy. This can result in issues such as:

- **Luteal Phase Defect**: A shortened luteal phase (less than 10 days) can mean that the uterine lining isn't properly maintained, making it difficult for an embryo to implant. This is a common cause of **early miscarriages**.

- **Difficulty Sustaining Pregnancy**: Even if fertilization and implantation occur, low progesterone levels can lead to early pregnancy loss, as the body may not be able to support the pregnancy during its critical early stages.

Women who experience recurrent miscarriages often have low progesterone levels. Fortunately, **progesterone supplementation** is a common treatment that can help support a healthy luteal phase and pregnancy in these cases.

3. Thyroid Hormones: The Metabolic Regulators

The **thyroid gland** is often overlooked when considering fertility, but it plays an essential role in regulating the body's metabolism and supporting reproductive health. Thyroid hormones, primarily **T3** and **T4**, regulate how your body uses energy and influence many processes, including the regulation of menstrual cycles and ovulation.

If your thyroid is out of balance—whether **underactive (hypothyroidism)** or **overactive (hyperthyroidism)**—it can throw off the delicate balance of reproductive hormones and make it harder to conceive.

Hypothyroidism (Underactive Thyroid)

Hypothyroidism occurs when the thyroid doesn't produce enough thyroid hormone. This can slow down many bodily functions, including those related to reproduction. Hypothyroidism is often linked to fertility problems such as:

- **Irregular Menstrual Cycles**: An underactive thyroid can cause prolonged or infrequent periods, making it difficult to predict ovulation or achieve regular cycles.

- **Anovulation**: Hypothyroidism can interfere with the normal release of eggs from the ovaries, leading to anovulation.

- **Elevated Prolactin Levels**: Hypothyroidism can cause elevated levels of **prolactin**, a hormone that interferes with ovulation by suppressing the normal secretion of **follicle-stimulating hormone (FSH)** and **luteinizing hormone (LH)**.

Women with untreated hypothyroidism may also have difficulty sustaining a pregnancy because thyroid hormones are crucial for fetal development, especially in the first trimester. Hypothyroidism can lead to **miscarriage** or **preterm labor** if not properly managed.

Hyperthyroidism (Overactive Thyroid)

On the flip side, **hyperthyroidism** is a condition where the thyroid gland produces too much thyroid hormone, leading to a hypermetabolic state. This condition can also disrupt fertility by:

- **Shortened Menstrual Cycles**: Hyperthyroidism can cause shorter, lighter periods, which may affect the timing and regularity of ovulation.

- **Weight Loss and Nutrient Deficiencies**: The increased metabolic rate in hyperthyroidism can lead to unintended weight loss, which may impact reproductive health. Additionally, the body may have trouble absorbing essential nutrients necessary for ovulation and pregnancy.

- **Increased Miscarriage Risk**: Women with hyperthyroidism have a higher risk of **miscarriage**, particularly if their thyroid hormone levels are not well controlled during pregnancy.

Hyperthyroidism also increases the levels of **sex hormone-binding globulin (SHBG)**, a protein that binds to estrogen and testosterone, reducing the availability of these hormones. This can lead to hormonal imbalances that disrupt the menstrual cycle and impair fertility.

The Role of Diet, Stress, and Lifestyle in Fertility Management

While fertility may seem like a purely biological function, research consistently shows that **lifestyle factors**—what we eat, how we move, how we handle stress—are powerful determinants of reproductive health. The choices you make in your daily life, from your diet to how you manage stress, can have a profound impact on your hormonal balance and fertility. In fact, numerous studies suggest that adopting healthier lifestyle habits can significantly improve fertility outcomes, particularly for women facing hormonal imbalances, such as those with **polycystic ovary syndrome (PCOS)** or **irregular menstrual cycles**.

The Mediterranean Diet and Fertility

One of the most well-researched diets in relation to fertility is the **Mediterranean-style diet**. This way of eating emphasizes **whole foods, healthy fats, lean proteins**, and an abundance of **fruits and vegetables**, all of which provide the body with the essential nutrients needed to support optimal hormonal health.

What Makes the Mediterranean Diet Fertility-Friendly?

- **Healthy fats**: The Mediterranean diet is rich in **monounsaturated fats**, particularly from sources like **olive oil, avocados**, and **nuts**. These fats are crucial for hormone production, including the production of **estrogen** and **progesterone**. Hormones are made from cholesterol, so consuming the right kinds of fats helps ensure that the body has the building blocks it needs to maintain hormonal balance.

- **Lean proteins**: Lean sources of protein, such as **fish, poultry, eggs**, and **legumes**, are staples of the Mediterranean diet. Protein is essential for cellular function and repair, but the specific emphasis on **omega-3 fatty acids** from fish, such as **salmon** and **mackerel**, is particularly beneficial for fertility. Omega-3s have been shown to reduce **inflammation** and support healthy blood flow to the reproductive organs, which can improve **ovarian function** and **egg quality**.

- **Fiber and whole grains**: Whole grains and fiber-rich foods like **vegetables**, **fruits**, and **legumes** help regulate **insulin levels** and prevent insulin resistance, a common issue in women with PCOS. Insulin resistance can lead to elevated **androgens** (male hormones), which disrupt ovulation and menstrual regularity. By stabilizing blood sugar levels, the Mediterranean diet helps reduce these hormonal imbalances.

- **Antioxidants**: Fruits and vegetables are packed with **antioxidants**, such as **vitamins C and E**, which protect eggs from oxidative stress. Oxidative stress can damage the quality of eggs, making it harder for them to fertilize and implant. Antioxidant-rich foods, like **berries**, **leafy greens**, and **tomatoes**, help support the health of your reproductive cells.

Research Supporting the Mediterranean Diet and Fertility

Multiple studies have supported the link between the Mediterranean diet and improved fertility outcomes. One study published in the journal **Human Reproduction** found that women who closely adhered to a Mediterranean-style diet had a significantly higher chance of becoming pregnant, both naturally and through **assisted reproductive technology (ART)**, compared to women who did not follow the diet as closely.

Another study from the **Harvard T.H. Chan School of Public Health** showed that women who followed a Mediterranean-style diet had a lower risk of developing ovulatory infertility. These findings are likely due to the diet's ability to support hormonal balance, reduce inflammation, and improve insulin sensitivity—all of which are key factors in reproductive health.

The Role of Stress Management in Fertility

While diet is a critical component of fertility, it's equally important to recognize the impact of **stress** on reproductive health. **Chronic stress** doesn't just affect your mental and emotional well-being; it can also wreak havoc on your hormones, leading to issues like **anovulation** (the absence of ovulation) and **irregular menstrual cycles**.

How Stress Disrupts Hormones

When you're under chronic stress, your body produces higher levels of **cortisol**, a stress hormone. Cortisol is part of the body's **fight-or-flight** response, and while it's useful in short bursts, ongoing elevated levels of cortisol can have a cascade of negative effects on your reproductive hormones:

- **Progesterone-steal phenomenon**: Cortisol and **progesterone** share a precursor hormone, and when the body is producing high levels of cortisol, it "steals" this precursor, leading to lower levels of progesterone. This can disrupt the second half of the menstrual cycle (the **luteal phase**) and make it difficult to maintain a healthy pregnancy.

- **Disruption of the hypothalamic-pituitary-ovarian (HPO) axis**: The HPO axis is responsible for regulating the menstrual cycle and ovulation. Chronic stress can disrupt the communication between these glands, leading to irregular cycles or anovulation.

Mind-Body Practices for Stress Reduction and Fertility

Research has shown that engaging in **mind-body practices**, such as **meditation**, **yoga**, and **deep breathing exercises**, can help reduce cortisol levels, improve hormonal balance, and increase the chances of conception.

1. Meditation and Mindfulness

Meditation, particularly **mindfulness-based stress reduction (MBSR)**, has been shown to significantly reduce stress and improve overall well-being. By regularly practicing mindfulness, women can lower their stress hormone levels, which in turn helps regulate their reproductive hormones. In one study, women undergoing **in vitro fertilization (IVF)** who participated in an MBSR program had higher rates of successful pregnancy compared to those who did not.

Meditation helps activate the **parasympathetic nervous system**, which is responsible for the body's "rest and digest" functions, allowing the body to move out of the chronic stress response and support more balanced hormone production.

2. Yoga

Yoga is another powerful tool for managing stress and supporting fertility. Yoga helps to relax the body and mind while also providing physical benefits such as improved circulation and flexibility. Certain yoga poses, such as those that focus on the **pelvic region**, are believed to increase blood flow to the reproductive organs and support the alignment of the pelvic muscles.

One study published in the journal **Fertility and Sterility** found that women who practiced yoga for just 45 minutes a day over a 6-week period had lower levels of cortisol and increased rates of ovulation. Yoga's combination of physical movement, controlled breathing, and mental relaxation makes it an effective way to reduce stress and support overall fertility.

3. Deep Breathing and Relaxation Techniques

Simple **deep breathing exercises** can have a profound impact on reducing stress. By taking slow, deep breaths, you stimulate the vagus nerve, which triggers the body's relaxation response and lowers cortisol levels. **Progressive muscle relaxation**, where you systematically tense and relax different muscle groups, can also help release tension from the body and reduce stress hormone production.

Weight Management and Fertility

Maintaining a **healthy weight** is another critical factor in supporting fertility, particularly for women with conditions like PCOS, where weight and insulin sensitivity are closely tied to hormonal balance.

Impact of Excess Weight on Fertility

Carrying excess weight, particularly around the abdomen, is associated with **insulin resistance**. Insulin resistance can lead to increased levels of androgens, which can interfere with ovulation and contribute to irregular menstrual cycles. Women with excess body fat may also experience **estrogen dominance**, where the body produces more estrogen than it needs, disrupting the balance of progesterone and estrogen.

Research has shown that losing even a small percentage of body weight (5-10%) can significantly improve **ovulatory function** and increase the likelihood of conception in women with PCOS or other hormonal imbalances.

Impact of Underweight on Fertility

On the flip side, being **underweight** can also negatively impact fertility. Women with a body mass index (BMI) below 18.5 often have low estrogen levels, which can prevent ovulation altogether. Conditions such as **hypothalamic amenorrhea**, where the hypothalamus slows or stops the release of reproductive hormones due to low body weight or excessive exercise, can make it difficult to conceive.

For women who are underweight, gaining weight through a balanced, nutrient-rich diet can restore regular menstrual cycles and improve chances of conception.

Conclusion: Lifestyle as a Pillar of Fertility

The connection between lifestyle factors and fertility is undeniable. A nutrient-dense diet, regular physical activity, and effective stress management not only support general health but are also key to optimizing reproductive function. The Mediterranean diet, with its emphasis on whole foods and healthy fats, provides the essential nutrients needed for hormonal balance and healthy ovulation. Meanwhile, mind-body practices like meditation and yoga help reduce stress, allowing the body to maintain a state of hormonal equilibrium that's conducive to conception.

By taking control of your lifestyle, you're not just improving your chances of conceiving; you're creating a foundation for long-term health and well-being for yourself and your future family.

Chapter 19

ADDRESSING COMMON MYTHS ABOUT HORMONAL HEALTH

WHEN IT COMES TO hormones, there is no shortage of misconceptions and myths that can lead to confusion, mismanagement, and unnecessary fear. Many people believe that hormones only play a role in reproduction or that hormone replacement therapy (HRT) is inherently dangerous. These myths can prevent individuals from taking the necessary steps to maintain or restore hormonal balance, especially when it comes to optimizing health at various stages of life.

In this chapter, we'll debunk some of the most common myths about hormonal health, clarify misunderstandings surrounding hormone replacement therapy, and explore how hormones are relevant far beyond just reproduction. My goal is to equip you with accurate, science-backed information so that you can make informed decisions about your hormonal health.

Myth 1: "Hormones Only Affect Reproduction"

One of the most prevalent myths about hormones is that they only play a role in reproductive functions, such as menstruation, pregnancy, and menopause. This couldn't be further from the truth. While it's true that hormones like **estrogen**, **progesterone**, and **testosterone** are critical for reproductive health, they also regulate many other bodily processes, impacting your overall well-being at every stage of life.

Hormones and Metabolism

Take **insulin**, for example. This hormone is crucial for regulating your blood sugar levels and plays a significant role in how your body metabolizes carbohydrates, fats, and proteins. Imbalances in insulin can lead to **insulin resistance**, a condition that increases the risk of developing **type 2 diabetes** and **metabolic syndrome**. This highlights how hormones are vital for metabolic health and energy regulation, far beyond reproduction.

Another critical hormone is **thyroid hormone**, which regulates your body's **metabolic rate**, **energy levels**, and **body temperature**. Whether you're a teenager or well into your 60s, thyroid hormones continue to affect your overall health. An underactive thyroid (**hypothyroidism**) can cause **weight gain**, **fatigue**, and **depression**, while an overactive thyroid (**hyperthyroidism**) can lead to **weight loss**, **anxiety**, and **insomnia**.

Hormones and Mental Health

Hormones also have a significant impact on mental health. **Cortisol**, commonly known as the "stress hormone," plays a key role in how your body responds to stress. Chronically elevated cortisol levels due to persistent stress can disrupt **sleep patterns, increase anxiety**, and even lead to **depression**. Additionally, hormones like **serotonin** and **dopamine** (neurotransmitters influenced by hormonal fluctuations) are directly tied to mood regulation. Estrogen, for example, influences serotonin production, which is why **menstrual cycle fluctuations, perimenopause**, and **menopause** can cause mood swings or even mood disorders.

Hormones and Bone Health

Estrogen isn't just a reproductive hormone; it also plays a vital role in maintaining **bone density**. As estrogen levels decline with age—especially during menopause—women face an increased risk of **osteoporosis** and bone fractures. Men also experience a gradual decline in **testosterone**, which affects both muscle mass and bone health.

So, hormones affect **everything from how your body processes food** to **how your brain regulates mood**, and they continue to be crucial at all stages of life.

Myth 2: "Hormone Replacement Therapy (HRT) Is Dangerous"

There's been a lot of controversy and misunderstanding surrounding **Hormone Replacement Therapy (HRT)**, particularly in women going through **menopause**. Many believe that HRT is dangerous and increases the risk of **breast cancer, heart disease**, or **blood**

clots. While it's true that HRT isn't without risks, it's essential to understand the context and the evolution of HRT treatments.

A Brief History of HRT and Risk Perception

Much of the fear surrounding HRT stems from the **Women's Health Initiative (WHI)** study in the early 2000s. This study raised concerns about the risks of long-term HRT use, particularly regarding **breast cancer** and **cardiovascular disease**. However, subsequent research has shown that the risks highlighted in the WHI study were somewhat overstated and didn't account for **different types of HRT**, **timing of use**, or **individual health profiles**.

For example, we now understand that the risks of HRT are largely dependent on **when** the therapy is initiated. Starting HRT earlier, particularly within the first 10 years of menopause, tends to show far fewer risks than starting it later in life. Moreover, newer formulations of HRT, such as **bioidentical hormones**, offer options that may carry fewer side effects than synthetic hormones.

Understanding the Risks and Benefits

While there are risks associated with HRT, these need to be weighed against its many benefits, particularly for women suffering from severe menopausal symptoms such as **hot flashes**, **night sweats**, **vaginal dryness**, and **osteoporosis**. HRT can significantly improve quality of life for women experiencing such symptoms.

Additionally, HRT may provide **cardiovascular protection** when started early in menopause, due to estrogen's positive effects on **blood vessels** and **cholesterol levels**. The risk of heart disease often rises after menopause, and early intervention with HRT can potentially mitigate some of this risk.

The Role of Bioidentical Hormones

Bioidentical hormones have gained popularity in recent years due to their ability to closely mimic the body's natural hormones. These hormones are chemically identical to the hormones produced by the body, making them a more "natural" option than synthetic hormones. Some believe bioidentical hormones are safer than traditional HRT, though more research is needed to confirm this.

Ultimately, the decision to use HRT should be made on a case-by-case basis in consultation with a healthcare provider. It's important to weigh the **risks and benefits** based on your health history, symptoms, and personal preferences. For many women, the benefits of symptom relief and improved quality of life far outweigh the risks when HRT is initiated at the appropriate time and with proper monitoring.

Myth 3: "Hormones Only Matter During Menstruation or Menopause"

Another common myth is that hormones are only important during specific life stages, like **puberty**, **menstruation**, or **menopause**. In reality, hormones are relevant throughout life and play a role in your health and well-being far beyond just reproductive phases.

Hormones in Youth and Adolescence

During **adolescence**, the body undergoes significant hormonal changes as the reproductive system matures. Both boys and girls experience surges in hormones like **estrogen** and **testosterone** during **puberty**, which trigger physical changes, emotional shifts, and the development of sexual characteristics.

However, hormonal imbalances during adolescence—such as in **PCOS** or **early onset hypothyroidism**—can lead to long-term health challenges. Early identification and management of these issues are essential for supporting hormonal health throughout life.

Hormones in Adulthood

Even in adulthood, beyond reproductive phases, your hormones continue to regulate essential processes like **metabolism, muscle mass**, and **mental clarity**. Hormones like **cortisol, insulin**, and **growth hormone** are crucial for maintaining **energy levels, body composition**, and **cognitive function**.

Testosterone continues to play a role in both men and women throughout adulthood. In men, testosterone helps maintain **muscle mass, bone density**, and **libido**. For women, testosterone (produced in smaller amounts) also contributes to **energy levels** and **sexual desire**. An imbalance in testosterone can lead to fatigue, weight gain, and reduced libido in both genders.

Hormones in Aging

As we age, hormonal levels naturally decline. However, these declines don't happen overnight, nor do they signal the end of hormonal health. In men, testosterone levels gradually decline, which can lead to **andropause**, a condition that includes symptoms like **fatigue**, **depression**, and **muscle loss**. In women, menopause marks the end of reproductive years, but hormones continue to influence **bone density**, **heart health**, and **mental health** long after menopause.

For both men and women, managing hormonal health as you age is crucial for maintaining **vitality**, **strength**, and **mental clarity**. Proper diet, exercise, stress management, and, in some cases, hormone therapies, can help mitigate the natural decline in hormones that comes with age.

Conclusion: Empowering Yourself with Knowledge

Hormonal health is far more nuanced than simply reproduction or managing symptoms during menopause. Your hormones regulate every aspect of your life—from how you store energy, to how you feel emotionally, to how well you sleep. Understanding the myths and realities of hormone balance is key to taking control of your health at every stage of life.

By debunking myths like "hormones only affect reproduction" and clarifying the role of HRT and bioidentical hormones, we empower ourselves to make informed decisions about our health. Hormones are relevant at all stages of life, and by understanding their complexities, you can proactively support your body, whether you're navigating adolescence, adulthood, or aging.

The goal is to take action—to balance your hormones with **diet**, **exercise**, **stress management**, and, when needed, medical interventions like HRT. With the right knowledge, you can navigate the often-confusing world of hormones with confidence and clarity.

Conclusion

The Path to Health, Longevity, and Hormonal Balance

Throughout this book, we've taken a deep dive into the critical role hormones play in your overall health. Hormonal balance isn't just a buzzword; it's a foundational aspect of wellness that affects every part of your life—from your physical health and emotional well-being to your longevity. Achieving hormonal balance requires understanding your body's unique signals and implementing lifestyle strategies that allow you to maintain it for the long term.

As you've learned, hormones are involved in virtually every process in the body. They regulate your metabolism, your mood, your reproductive health, and your immune system. When your hormones are in balance, you feel energized, strong, and emotionally stable. But when they're out of balance, even seemingly small disruptions can lead to a cascade of symptoms, from fatigue and weight gain to anxiety, depression, and reduced cognitive function. The path to health and longevity lies in managing and optimizing these hormones so they work for you, not against you.

Let's take a moment to reflect on the most important takeaways from this book and how you can implement the strategies discussed to achieve lasting health, vitality, and hormonal balance.

Why Hormonal Balance is Critical for Overall Well-Being

Your body's hormonal system is like a symphony, with each hormone playing a crucial role. When all of the instruments—your **cortisol**, **estrogen**, **progesterone**, **thyroid hormones**, **insulin**, and others—are in harmony, your body functions optimally. But when even one hormone is out of balance, it can throw off the entire system, resulting in a range of issues that affect your day-to-day life.

1. Physical Well-Being

At its core, hormonal balance is about keeping your body functioning as it should. Hormones regulate your metabolism, control how your body stores and uses fat, and determine your energy levels. When you experience **insulin resistance**, for example, your body struggles to use glucose effectively, which can lead to weight gain, fatigue, and an increased risk of chronic conditions like **type 2 diabetes** and **heart disease**.

Similarly, hormones like **cortisol** and **thyroid hormones** are key to regulating your energy and metabolism. If your cortisol levels are chronically elevated due to stress, your body may store fat more easily, especially around your midsection, while also disrupting your sleep patterns. **Thyroid hormones**, on the other hand, help control your metabolic rate—so if you have **hypothyroidism**, you may experience sluggishness, weight gain, and low energy levels. When hormones like these are in balance, your body can manage stress, burn energy efficiently, and keep your weight in check.

2. Emotional and Mental Health

Your hormones don't just affect your physical health—they also have a profound impact on your mood, cognition, and overall mental well-being. **Estrogen** and **progesterone**, for example, are closely linked to your emotional state. Fluctuations in these hormones can contribute to **mood swings**, **irritability**, **anxiety**, and even **depression**. This is why many women experience emotional turbulence during **premenstrual syndrome (PMS)**, **perimenopause**, and **menopause**, when these hormone levels are in flux.

On a daily basis, hormones like **cortisol** and **serotonin** regulate how you respond to stress and how happy or calm you feel. When these hormones are out of balance, it can lead to symptoms of **depression**, **chronic anxiety**, and **burnout**. Proper hormonal balance ensures you have the emotional resilience to handle life's challenges and feel a sense of calm and stability in your everyday life.

3. Longevity and Disease Prevention

Maintaining balanced hormones is also a key factor in promoting longevity and preventing disease. Hormonal imbalances can increase the risk of developing **chronic conditions** such as **heart disease, osteoporosis**, and **cognitive decline**. For example, as **estrogen** levels decline during menopause, women are at higher risk of developing **osteoporosis** and **cardiovascular disease** due to the protective role estrogen plays in bone density and heart health. Similarly, **testosterone** levels in men, when diminished, can contribute to the loss of muscle mass, energy, and libido, and can also affect mood and cognitive function.

The good news is that taking steps to restore hormonal balance can significantly reduce the risk of these conditions. By focusing on holistic lifestyle changes—such as improving your diet, incorporating regular exercise, managing stress, and optimizing sleep—you can not only restore hormonal balance but also promote long-term health and vitality.

Implementing Strategies for Lasting Health and Vitality

Now that you have a deeper understanding of the critical role hormones play in your health, it's time to take action. Achieving hormonal balance requires consistent, intentional effort. The strategies outlined in this book aren't quick fixes; they are long-term lifestyle changes designed to support your body's natural ability to regulate hormones and maintain equilibrium.

1. Focus on Nutrient-Dense, Hormone-Supporting Foods

Your diet is one of the most powerful tools you have for regulating your hormones. The foods you eat provide the building blocks your body needs to produce and balance hormones. By focusing on a diet rich in whole, nutrient-dense foods, you can directly support your hormonal health.

- **Healthy Fats**: Include foods like **avocados**, **olive oil**, **nuts**, and **fatty fish** (such as salmon) in your diet to provide the essential fats needed for hormone production. Fats are crucial for the synthesis of hormones like **estrogen**, **progesterone**, and **testosterone**.

- **Protein**: Ensure you're getting enough high-quality protein from sources like **eggs**, **lean meats**, **legumes**, and **quinoa**. Protein provides the amino acids your body uses to create enzymes and hormones, which regulate many bodily functions, including metabolism and mood.

- **Fiber and Whole Grains**: High-fiber foods like **vegetables**, **fruits**, and **whole grains** help maintain healthy blood sugar levels, reduce insulin resistance, and support the elimination of excess hormones. Fiber can also aid in digestion and prevent constipation, which is vital for detoxifying excess estrogen.

- **Antioxidants**: Foods rich in antioxidants, such as **berries**, **leafy greens**, and **nuts**, protect your cells from damage caused by oxidative stress and inflammation, which can disrupt hormone production and balance.

In addition to these nutrient-dense foods, it's essential to limit processed foods, added sugars, and unhealthy fats, all of which can trigger inflammation, insulin resistance, and hormonal imbalances.

2. Manage Stress to Lower Cortisol Levels

Stress is one of the biggest disruptors of hormonal balance, particularly through the overproduction of **cortisol**, the body's primary stress hormone. Chronic stress leads to **cortisol dysregulation**, which can result in weight gain, disrupted sleep, increased cravings, and a weakened immune system.

To reduce stress and keep cortisol levels in check, incorporate stress-reducing activities into your daily routine:

- **Mindfulness and Meditation**: Practicing mindfulness, meditation, or even simple deep breathing exercises can help activate your parasympathetic nervous system (the "rest and digest" system) and lower cortisol levels.

- **Yoga and Gentle Movement**: Gentle forms of exercise, such as yoga or tai chi, not only reduce stress but also support hormone balance by improving circulation and promoting relaxation.

- **Time in Nature**: Spending time outdoors, especially in natural settings like parks, forests, or near bodies of water, can significantly lower stress hormones and improve mental clarity.

By focusing on stress management techniques, you can prevent cortisol from wreaking havoc on your hormonal system and help restore balance.

3. Prioritize Sleep for Optimal Hormonal Health

Sleep is one of the most powerful, yet often overlooked, factors in maintaining hormonal balance. During sleep, your body repairs and restores itself, and many hormones—like **growth hormone** and **melatonin**—are regulated during deep sleep cycles. **Poor sleep** or **chronic sleep deprivation** can disrupt hormones like **cortisol**, **insulin**, and **ghrelin** (the hunger hormone), leading to weight gain, fatigue, and increased stress.

To improve your sleep quality:

- **Establish a Consistent Sleep Routine**: Go to bed and wake up at the same time each day, even on weekends. Consistency helps regulate your body's internal clock (circadian rhythm).

- **Create a Sleep-Friendly Environment**: Keep your bedroom cool, dark, and quiet to promote restful sleep. Avoid screens and blue light exposure before bed, as these can interfere with melatonin production.

- **Practice Relaxation Before Bed**: Engaging in calming activities, such as reading, taking a warm bath, or practicing meditation, can help signal to your body that it's time to wind down.

By making sleep a priority, you support not only your energy levels but also the hormonal systems that regulate everything from appetite to stress.

4. Stay Active for Long-Term Health

Exercise is one of the best ways to maintain hormonal balance, particularly when it comes to regulating hormones like **insulin**, **estrogen**, **testosterone**, and **growth hormone**. Regular physical activity helps lower cortisol levels, improve insulin sensitivity, and maintain a healthy weight, all of which are key factors in hormonal health.

- **Strength Training**: Incorporating strength training exercises, such as weightlifting or resistance bands, helps build lean muscle mass, which supports the production of testosterone and growth hormone, both of which decline with age.

- **Cardio and HIIT**: Cardiovascular exercise, whether it's walking, jogging, or high-intensity interval training (HIIT), improves insulin sensitivity and cardiovascular health, both of which are essential for managing hormones like insulin and cortisol.

- **Flexibility and Mobility**: Incorporating activities that improve flexibility and mobility, such as yoga or Pilates, not only help relieve stress but also support circulation and overall hormonal health.

By staying active and making movement a part of your daily routine, you can optimize your hormone levels and promote long-term health.

The Long-Term Path to Hormonal Balance and Well-Being

Achieving hormonal balance is not an overnight process. It requires dedication, consistency, and a holistic approach that addresses every aspect of your health—from what you eat and how you move to how you manage stress and sleep. The strategies outlined in this book are designed to give you the tools you need to optimize your hormone levels and feel your best, no matter what stage of life you're in.

Remember, your hormones are not static; they fluctuate in response to your environment, lifestyle, and aging process. But by taking proactive steps to support your body's natural processes, you can enjoy a life full of vitality, energy, and balance.

The journey to hormonal balance is a lifelong one, but the rewards—better health, improved mood, and greater longevity—are well worth the effort. You've already taken the first step by educating yourself, and now it's time to put that knowledge into action.

Glossary of Terms

Key Terms Related to Hormones and Health

1. Adrenal Glands

Small glands located on top of each kidney that produce hormones such as **cortisol** and **adrenaline**. These hormones help regulate stress responses, metabolism, and immune function.

2. Androgens

A group of hormones, including **testosterone**, is typically higher in males but also present in females. They play a role in reproductive health, libido, and muscle mass.

3. Bioidentical Hormones

Hormones that are chemically identical to those produced by the human body. Commonly used in **Hormone Replacement Therapy (HRT)**, bioidentical hormones are designed to mimic natural hormones like **estrogen** and **progesterone**.

4. Cortisol

Often referred to as the "stress hormone," **cortisol** is produced by the adrenal glands and helps regulate the body's response to stress, controls metabolism, and maintains blood sugar levels.

5. Endocrine System

A network of glands and organs that produce, store, and release hormones. The endocrine system regulates many bodily functions, including metabolism, growth, and reproduction.

6. Estrogen

A primary female sex hormone responsible for the development and regulation of the female reproductive system, including the menstrual cycle and pregnancy. It also plays a role in bone health, mood regulation, and fat distribution.

7. Follicle-stimulating hormone (FSH)

A hormone produced by the **pituitary gland** that stimulates the growth of ovarian follicles in women and the production of sperm in men.

8. Hypothyroidism

A condition in which the thyroid gland produces too little **thyroid hormone**, leading to symptoms like weight gain, fatigue, and depression.

9. Insulin

A hormone produced by the **pancreas** that regulates blood sugar by allowing cells to absorb glucose. **Insulin resistance** occurs when the body's cells don't respond properly to insulin, leading to elevated blood sugar levels.

10. Luteal Phase

The second half of the menstrual cycle after ovulation, during which the hormone **progesterone** prepares the uterus for possible pregnancy. If pregnancy does not occur, **progesterone** levels drop, triggering menstruation.

11. Progesterone

A hormone involved in the menstrual cycle and pregnancy. It prepares the uterine lining for implantation and helps maintain pregnancy. Low progesterone levels can lead to **menstrual irregularities** or difficulty maintaining pregnancy.

12. Testosterone

A primary male sex hormone that is also present in women in smaller amounts. In men, it regulates libido, muscle mass, and sperm production. In women, it plays a role in sexual desire and energy levels.

13. Thyroid Gland

A gland located in the neck that produces **thyroid hormones** (T3 and T4), which regulate metabolism, energy levels, and body temperature.

14. Thyroid Hormones (T3 and T4)

Hormones produced by the **thyroid gland** that regulate the body's metabolism, energy production, and many other functions. Imbalances can lead to conditions like **hypothyroidism** or **hyperthyroidism**.

15. Xenoestrogens

Synthetic compounds found in plastics, cosmetics, and certain foods that mimic the hormone **estrogen** in the body. Exposure to xenoestrogens can lead to hormonal imbalances, including **estrogen dominance**.

Dear Reader,

THANK YOU SO MUCH for taking the time to read this book! If you found it helpful, inspiring, or enjoyable in any way, I would be truly grateful if you could take a moment to leave a positive review on Amazon or any other site where you love to share your thoughts.

Your reviews help other readers discover this book and let them know how it might benefit them as well. More importantly, your feedback allows me to continue writing and sharing more content that can hopefully make a positive impact in others' lives.

Every review makes a huge difference—whether it's a few sentences or a detailed account of your experience. It would mean the world to me, and I sincerely appreciate your support!

With gratitude,
Alexandra Hart

Other Books by Alexandra Hart

If you found this book helpful, you might enjoy exploring some of my other works. Each book is designed to provide practical insights and tools for personal growth, healing, and emotional well-being.

1. **I'm So F*cking Depressed All The Time: A Psychiatrist's Unfiltered Journey Through Depression**

2. **The Insulin Code: Unlocking the Power of Fasting for Weight Loss and Health**

3. **The Sugar Code: Breaking Free from Sugar Addiction for Better Health and Diabetes Control**

4. **Breaking Free from Relationship Anxiety: A Journey to Healing Anxious-Preoccupied Attachment**

5. **The Emotional Intelligence Handbook: Practical Strategies to Enhance Your Relationships, Career, and Well-Being**

6. **The Healing Legacy: Breaking the Chains of Generational Trauma**

7. **Breaking Free: A Journey to Overcoming Narcissistic Abuse**

8. **28-Day Fasting Journey: A Supportive Guide to Achieving Health, Weight Loss, and Mental Clarity for Beginners**

9. **Healing Your Inner Child Workbook: A Comprehensive Guide to Overcoming Childhood Wounds, Building Self-Compassion, and Reclaiming Your Life (For Adults)**

10. **Her Voice, Her Power: Essays on Feminism, Identity, and the Fight for Equality: Amplifying Women's Stories Across Cultures and Generations (Empowerment and Healing: A Journey to Mental Wellness**

11. **Achieve Your Dreams: The Ultimate Guide to Goal Setting and Achievement**

12. **Embracing Love: A Parent's Guide to Supporting and Empowering LGBTQ+ Children with Compassion and Confidence**

About Alexandra Hart

Alexandra Hart is a dedicated psychiatrist with a passion for understanding the complexities of the human mind and fostering mental well-being. With years of experience in the field, Alexandra has worked extensively with individuals from diverse backgrounds, helping them navigate life's challenges and achieve emotional balance. Her approach to psychiatry is deeply rooted in empathy, evidence-based practices, and a commitment to holistic care.

Driven by a desire to make mental health resources accessible and relatable, Alexandra has contributed to various mental health initiatives and projects, sharing her insights on topics such as emotional resilience, personal growth, and the importance of self-care. Her work reflects a profound understanding of the interconnectedness of mental health, identity, and overall well-being.

In her free time, Alexandra enjoys exploring the arts, engaging in thoughtful discussions, and continuously learning about the ever-evolving field of psychiatry. She is passionate about helping others lead fulfilling lives and is dedicated to making a positive impact on the mental health landscape.

To read more books from the author and join her community, you can scan the code below, or go to the link – https://substack.com/@alexandrahart1

Printed in Great Britain
by Amazon